Woman Who Loves A Dog

CATHERINE A. HOSMER

iUniverse, Inc.
New York   Bloomington

Woman Who Loves A Dog

The views expressed in this work are solely those of the author and do not necessarily reflect the views of the publisher, and the publisher hereby disclaims any responsibility for them.

iUniverse books may be ordered through booksellers or by contacting:

iUniverse
1663 Liberty Drive
Bloomington, IN 47403
www.iuniverse.com
1-800-Authors (1-800-288-4677)

Because of the dynamic nature of the Internet, any Web addresses or links contained in this book may have changed since publication and may no longer be valid.

ISBN: 978-1-4502-1456-8 (sc)
ISBN: 978-1-4502-1457-5 (ebk)

Printed in the United States of America

iUniverse rev. date: 6/4/2010

DEDICATED TO PUCK

AND HIS SKILLED AND KIND VETERINARIANS

CHAPTER ONE

When I was 17, I knew that I was fat. It was perfectly obvious. I stood on the scale and even if it said only 87 pounds, I knew it was wrong. And even if it was right, when I stood before a mirror, I could see how fat I was--that my stomach bulged and my arms were too flabby and my legs--ugh!--how could they be so thick, and not curvy and slim like those pictures of girls in magazines? Did boys like me? Not a chance. I was a basket case with boys. My friends tried to convince me that I was too thin, but I told them I wasn't thin enough, that was the trouble and even they didn't believe me. One told me right out that I ought to see a shrink. Talk to your dad, she said, he's a doctor and knows about this. It's called bulimia, kiddo, my sister had it, and you've got it bad.

So I began to stay away from friends who obviously didn't know anything, and I kept to my room more and more. I studied, but I always got the best marks in the class anyway without studying so why worry. One of my teachers became alarmed about how thin I was, and even sent a note home to my mother suggesting I get help. That teacher meant well and I really liked her. She taught math and I was always a whiz at math so she took me under her wing. My father, a doctor, wanted me to see a shrink. I didn't want to see a shrink. What would he know? I mean I knew I was all right, that when I finally got thin enough I'd stop heading off to the john to upchuck my meals. But I had a lot of weight to lose before then.

My Dad came to my room one night and said, "Amy, you've got to stop this. You've got to get help. You're wasting away to nothing and I can't help you. I'm alarmed and your mother's about out of her mind. Let me take you to Barsamian—he's a good psychiatrist and you need help. Do you hear me, darling? I mean it."

He's gone all the time. He wanted me to be a doctor, especially after my brother, Brian, was killed in Iraq. Brian wanted to be a doctor. No way am I going to be a doctor. I'd never be a doctor. Gone all night and day, that's a life?

For some reason my classmates ignore me, but make comments about my weight. "Toothpick," they call me, and "Skinny Bean." It doesn't bother me. They don't know how really fat I look in my mirror every morning. Wait until they see me when I get thin. In school I eat a normal lunch every day, then beat it to the bathroom to upchuck. They have no idea what I'm doing, except I think that Ruth, my best friend, has an inkling. During gym weigh-ins I weighed less than any girl in my class, and I'm not about to jeopardize that. I'm not going to be fat. Not me.

Ruth almost gave up on me. "You're way over your head, Amy," she said to me one day. "What are you trying to do to yourself? Frankly, you look like a skeleton. I can see every bone in your body. I walk home with you every day after school, and all you want to do is crawl into bed."

"No, I wake up and study." What does Ruth know?

"That's a life?"

I had a moment of truth and since she's my best friend, I talk to her more than anyone else. "Sometimes I want to die, Ruth."

Then she grabbed me around the shoulders and shook me, hard. Every bone in my body rattled. "Don't you dare talk like that, Amy. You're not going to die. I'm not going to let you, you hear me? Amy, wake up. Sometimes you scare me half to death."

"I'm sorry, but..."

"But what? Don't you see what you're doing? Is this because your brother died? I know how much you loved him, but is your grief worth this, hurting yourself? Haven't you suffered enough? Haven't your parents suffered enough? You've got to stop..."

"Don't yell at me!" I answered, yelling back. Once I lost the fat across my butt, I'd start eating again. Ruth didn't know that but I did. When I look in my mirror after my shower every morning, I still see that revolting layer covering my thighs and hips. When I started to tell this to Ruth, she didn't want to hear it. Then I knew I was on my own.

I kept thinking about my brother, Brian, who was the person I cared about most in the world, except for my parents. An older brother is a dream, every girl wants one, and not necessarily to bring boys home, but that counts for something, too. He was so wonderful, so cool. I could tell my secrets to him and he wouldn't even laugh. I think about him all the time, and soak my pillow with my tears at night. As kids we'd argued and wrestled, and I threw pillows at him and called him a dork, and he laughed at me and told me to grow up. He was handsome as a movie star so the girls were always calling his cell. Even Ruth said he was terrific.

Oh why, why wasn't he here now? What good did it do that he went to that miserable place? My stomach hurts every time I think about him, blown apart in that stinking desert. I told him not to go to Iraq. I insisted, I cried and pleaded, saying that it was a stupid thing to do. Didn't he know that people got killed in Iraq, and that I'd die if something happened to him? He was my very own brother. But he just smiled with a faraway expression in his eyes and said that it was his duty to go. I said, what the hell is duty, nobody was pushing him to go, that it was just crazy.

"Please don't go," I'd pleaded. "I know that I get obnoxious sometimes, but I won't kid you anymore if you stay home."

"Listen, little sis," he said, putting his arm around my shoulder, "I'm gonna come back in one piece, you wait and see. You don't have to worry." He said that he had to go and I said no, you don't. We argued for a month before he left, and I sobbed that whole month. He hadn't been in Iraq for six months when he stepped on a land mine, blowing himself up along with two of his buddies.

I remember the officer coming to the door. I could see his mouth move but I stopped hearing his words. I stuffed my fingers in my ears, hating what he was saying. My parents seemed to turn inside out, listening to him. It was plain agony. I couldn't look at them, but I grabbed my mother around the neck and shook with sobs.

Brian wasn't coming back, ever. I'd never see him again, never talk to him, never tell him jokes or kid him about his girlfriends? His body was blown to pieces!

Why did he ever go to that awful place? It was so useless. I told him, I warned him. What did he get from it? What did we get from it? My beautiful, beautiful brother, gone forever.

Afterward, I went to bed and didn't want to get up, ever again. I wanted to go to sleep and never wake up. Finally Dad did put me in the hospital when I didn't eat, and hauled me off to a shrink. I bet that shrink never lost a brother. He didn't even understand, he'd never understand.

My legs hurt all the time and the school doctor said I was losing muscle mass. I hadn't had a period in months, which really didn't bother me even if all the girls in my class talked about theirs as if now they were mature. I didn't feel womanly but I didn't care.

But summer vacation was soon coming and I would be left at home more often, left to myself and not be nagged to eat.

"What are you going to do all summer?" Ruth asked. "Stay in bed all day, Amy?"

"Of course not," I answered. "I'll get a summer job."

"Doing what?"

"Like you, maybe get work at a summer camp."

Ruth looked at me doubtfully. "How? Do you know how thin you are?"

I didn't want to argue with her. She was my best friend. And she didn't know how sore my legs and arms felt. I didn't want anyone to know. I even knew a summer camp was out of the question.

One day my grandparents, who spend a few months every summer visiting relatives, dropped by with Molly, their border collie, and asked my parents to look after her while they were away. My parents said, "Sure, she's a nice dog, we'll be glad to watch her." So a brown and white dog came to live with us for a few weeks. She was a run-of-the-mill mutt as far as I was concerned and it seemed as if she was going to be around forever.

My mother said, "Your father will be busy at the hospital much of the time, Amy, and I've got a busy week at the library. Can you manage to let Molly out after school? I'll try to make it home for lunch whenever I can."

The library was where Mom worked all day. I nodded but didn't have any intention of letting the mutt out. I was starting to feel pretty weak and I didn't want my parents to know that I was having a hard time getting to school every day, even though it was only two blocks away. I didn't want my father to put me in the hospital again. In the hospital I had gained two pounds and my father was so pleased that I was afraid he'd put me there again.

The first afternoon after school, I was in bed when I heard a noise on my mattress, a queer scratching. I peered over the edge, and there was the mutt, her eyes full and pleading.

"Go away," I said. "Can't you see I'm sleeping? Leave me alone, you stupid dog."

But Molly didn't take the hint. She didn't act as if she even heard me. When she scratched against the mattress again, I looked over the edge into a pair of wide brown liquid eyes. I remember what Mom had asked, that I was here alone with her. "I supposed you've got to go out," I said, groaning inwardly. "Why don't you just go away?"

But she obviously wasn't about to go away. Resigned, I reached for my robe and dragged myself to the front door. "Now go out," I said. "Scat! Beat it, you stupid mutt."

When Molly went to the door, she sat looking at me and wagging her tail. "You've got to be crazy," I told her, "if you think I'm going out with you."

She wouldn't leave the door, and I didn't want her peeing on the rug, so I finally took my school clothes out of the closet, put them back on, and walked her into the back yard, which was surrounded by a fence to keep groundhogs out of my father's garden. That dog was going to be the end of me. What did we need a dog for? Just how long did my grandparents expect us to watch her? "Go do your thing," I commanded, "so I can go back to bed."

She took her time, racing around the yard with sheer joy at being loose. Round and 'round she went, circling the fence like a maniac, legs flying, only stopping now and then for a shake. Her hair flew. I wished vaguely that I could summon her energy and joy of living.

I watched her, waiting impatiently for her to get ready to come back into the house. Did she think I was going to stand out there all day?

But the fresh air felt good. It actually smelled sweet, and I realized that Mom's lilacs were in bloom. I breathed in the marvelous scent,

5

feeling the moving air, seeing the buds on the trees turning pale green. I wondered for the first time why I was so sick. It was good to be thin, wasn't it? I acknowledged for the first time that I was really sick.

I knew it had something to do with a lack of proper food. But how could I get thinner and at the same time eat more food to make my legs and arms feel stronger? I couldn't answer my own question.

When Mom came home, I was trying to study while the dog slept by my desk, as if she thought I wanted her there. She'd wake up, lick her paws, then look at me. What did she expect? "Go back to sleep and leave me alone," I told her.

Mom said, "Amy, did you let Molly out? She certainly looks full of beans, as if she's had some exercise."

"She ran around the fence," I answered. "Several times."

She looked me over. "And you've got a little color in your cheeks. I bet it was good for you, too."

"My legs hurt," I answered. "It hurts to let her out."

"Well, thanks, darling. Grandma and Pop will be awfully pleased. They dote on that little dog."

I didn't care how much they doted on Molly. "When are they coming home? Do I have to take care of her every day?"

Mom shook her head. "I'll be here every weekend and sometimes during the week, too. When it isn't so busy at the library, I'll try to get home for lunch."

Well, she didn't make it home for lunch except twice, so I let the mutt out every day. Ruth came by most days after school and said that she thought Molly was cute. "Then you take her out," I said. "She's a pain. She thinks I'm her buddy."

"Well, you are, in a way." Ruth looked me over. "You look better, Amy. Really. Are you feeling better?"

I thought about it. "A little." Tell the truth, those outings with Molly made my breathing easier. I'd been taking her on a leash for walks down the street to the end of the block and back. She obviously loved it, bouncing along before me with spurts of energy and sniffing every tree in sight.

"I don't know what you're doing, Amy," Ruth said, "but it agrees with you. Your face looks fuller"

"I'm getting fat. I gained three pounds."

"Good! Please don't stop. I love you. You're my best friend. You need to gain more pounds. Please believe me."

I thought about it. This last week my legs had stopped aching so badly. And I didn't mind so much now if Molly wanted to go out. Maybe it wouldn't hurt walking the dog and trying to put on a couple more pounds. Not many, of course, maybe just two or three. But I found the idea scary. Why, I wondered, would walking Molly seem scary? Then I realized it wasn't walking the dog, which frightened me; it was gaining the pounds.

I looked at myself in the mirror. Already I could see the extra weight, or I thought I could. Did those pounds make me look fat? Well, not yet. I could stand a little more bosom because I was flat as a pancake. Even those skinny models had breasts, and maybe a boy would notice, 'though I didn't care much what boys thought.

"When are Grandma and Pops coming back from Ohio?" I asked Mom one day. "They're going to stay forever?"

"Next week," Mom said. "They've had a wonderful time."

"Then they can take back their mutt," I said. But I felt badly calling Molly a "mutt." She was even sleeping in my bed now, and I rubbed her ears before I went to sleep. She stopped my nightmares and I couldn't think about Brian so much. Maybe I'd even miss her.

My grandparents arrived over the next weekend. My grandmother exclaimed over me. "You look so much better, darling. You were absolutely skin and bones when we left. We were frightened for you."

"Now you can take Molly home," I said, looking down at the dog, which was sitting on my foot.

"We wouldn't think of it," Grandma said. "Your mother said she adores you. Just look at her. She won't leave your side. Besides, she's too much for us old folks."

"But..."

"She's saved your life," my mother added, more firmly than I'd ever heard her speak before. "Why you've gained ten pounds and look like a new person."

"I know, but I don't want to gain any more pounds. I mean it."

My grandparents departed, leaving Molly behind. She slept in my bed from then on. I walked her every day. Eventually we began running along a path through the woods, which Molly loved. I did, too. Her eyes gleamed when I picked up her leash. I fluffed the ruff around her neck and called her a good dog.

"Your Mom was right," Ruth said one day. "That little dog did save your life, Amy. You're a new person. I can hardly believe it. She's a little miracle dog, that's what she is."

I looked at Molly, sitting at my feet. "I know," I answered. "I suppose you're right."

"I *know* I'm right. Your parents do, too. That's why your grandparents gave you the dog. And because they can't manage a dog anymore."

I looked at her. "How do you know all this?"

"Because your Mom told me one day when I was here. She's right, too. I'm so glad. I prayed for you."

I thought then, in a moment of awareness, in a stab of insight, how lucky I was to have people who cared about me. I think they did save my life. I reached down to pet Molly once more.

CHAPTER TWO

Ruth and I decided to go to the same college, two hundred miles away. It was instate, not as expensive as most out-of-state schools, and we could come home on some weekends. Centerville, the town where I live in Florida, is a medium-size burg, with two main drags, small streets going off from the central park like spokes, a library, two shopping centers, a hospital, and a smattering of small businesses. The state university was huge, but that didn't bother me; my high school in Centerville had been large. I still wanted to hide myself and a big school was just about right. It happened that Ruth lived in the dorm next to mine and we attended a couple of the same classes.

"What are you taking?" she asked me the day we signed up.

"Biology, comparative anatomy, and physics, in addition to all the required classes."

"Why so many science courses? You'll spend all your time in labs."

"I don't care. They interest me."

She glanced at me. "What if you want to date? I heard that some of those courses have labs on weekends. You'll be all tied up."

"I'm not dating, so what difference does it make? I need lab hours."

"Why? You're not thinking of becoming a doctor, are you? To take your brother's place?"

I shook my head. "I don't want to be a doctor. Not like my Dad, anyway."

"Then what…"

"I think I might become a vet, Ruth. I've been looking into it."

"A…?"

"A veterinarian."

"You're serious? I can't believe it, Amy. You never told me."

"A dog saved my life, Ruth. You said so yourself. She's become special to me so I'd like to give it a try."

"But it'll take forever."

"They have a combined degree of general science and veterinary medicine here. So it won't take so long."

Ruth thought about it for a minute. "Well, you've got the marks for it. You can always change your mind."

I was pretty sure I wouldn't change my mind. I'd been thinking about becoming a vet ever since reading the university's curriculum and discovering you could take veterinary medicine beginning sophomore year. That meant that I could shorten the length of time I'd be in school by two years. I'd even mentioned it to Dad.

He'd put his arm around me. "You don't have to be a medical doctor like me, Amy," he said. "You don't have to fulfill Brian's ambition, either. If you decide you want to be a vet, your mother and I are behind you." My mother told me the same thing the next day. "It would be a fascinating career, Amy. I think you have a way with animals. Look how devoted Molly is to you."

It was true. I still worried about a return to bulimia but I'd experienced only one episode in a year, a miracle to my way of thinking. That occurred my senior high school year when a boy who sat next to me in my high school math class began talking to me. He was smart, good-looking and I got a crush on him. I thought he liked me, too. Then he began to date another girl and I cried and felt bulimic all over again. But I clung to Molly, burrowing my face in her soft coat, and told her all about it. I got over it then although I still worried it could come back. But I decided not to put my life on hold.

"Are you still thinking about nursing?" I asked Ruth.

Ruth nodded. "You know that Mom's a nurse. She's really tickled I'm going into her field. She says it's a lot easier now to get a job in nursing than in some other fields. Besides, I've been thinking about nursing for a while, so I thought I'd try it out."

I admired Ruth so much: she'd make a wonderful nurse. She was a naturally caring person. She'd restored my faith in myself in high school, along with Molly and my parents, while I was still gorging and purging. It was awful. I really did think I might die of my affliction. It still terrified me, because I know now how really sick I was and I didn't want to ever return to those days again.

To help make up my mind, I took out books about veterinary medicine from the library where Mom worked to see what professionals said about their own profession. Maybe I could get some advice. One of the books had been written by a veterinary surgeon at the very university I'm attending; another related the experiences of a doctor at the famous Angell Animal Medical Center in Boston, Dr. Havletic. His specialty: really serious animal injuries. He was incredible. He'd removed a butcher knife from a dog's stomach (How it got there, I couldn't imagine). He'd retrieved a bride's engagement ring from a dog's stomach the night before the couple's wedding; reattached a cat's face; treated snakes with throat problems (did he use l-o-n-g forceps?); and once operated on a dog with stomach pains and removed from his innards a pair of red panties, which didn't even belong to the owner. He'd cured goldfish, hamsters, turtles, and birds. I was fascinated.

Other doctors I read about had operated on iguanas, pythons, bobcats, beavers, and turtles. To me, it was unbelievable. I couldn't imagine how anyone could operate on a goldfish, or a hamster. One vet operated on a kid's pet rat. But when I read that parakeets were the third most popular pet in the United States, and that their heartbeats could go to six or seven hundred beats per minute merely by touching them, often leading to cardiac arrest, I began to doubt my choice of careers. I had a long way to go, but then and there I forswore ever treating a parakeet. But it was easy for me to have empathy for all the animals I read about, except maybe the rats and pythons.

Unfortunately, some doctors had to care for animals tortured and mistreated by humans, healing gunshot wounds as well as burns and lacerations. I simply couldn't imagine a human mistreating an animal although I'd read about it often enough in newspapers. What were these sick humans thinking? Why were they taking out their aggression on helpless animals? I'd heard that criminals often started their lives of sadistic crime by victimizing animals. I don't know how I'd react to an owner who'd deliberately injured an animal, but I knew I'd be furious. I couldn't bear to think of a kind dog like Molly being abused. But I'd have to put sick animals to sleep, and that would make me suffer as well. I didn't know if I could do it. I was going to have to be strong if I intended to enter this profession, and so far I'd been pretty much of a weakling.

I knew I couldn't specialize in large animal medicine because I could vividly picture a sick horse looking me straight in the eye as I attempted to treat it and wondering what I thought I was doing. Or birthing a cow, with my entire arm shoved up into the poor animal's birth canal trying to perform a maneuver I couldn't even see. No, I'd stick to the smaller of God's creatures even if some of their anatomies were minute and positively weird.

I also read that women had a hard time securing a place in veterinary school until thirty years ago. In fact, they were ostracized, just as they were in architecture, law, medical practice and practically every other professional field. This, in spite of the fact that female veterinarians had been around for over one hundred years. In 1903, I read, a lady named Mignon Nicholson became the first vet in the United States, although a woman named Aleen Cust preceded her admission to veterinarian college by nine years in England. Whereupon the Royal Veterinary College refused to give her a license to practice so she could never exercise her profession. I felt sorry for Dr. Cust: to go so far and then be rejected in her life's goal.

But one open-minded American doctor named Dr. Nick Trout came to the aid of woman vets when he wrote, "Cows may, in fact, prefer a delicate feminine arm up their bottom to that of some juiced Neanderthal, and besides, the 1960s ensured that women could trade their bra for a pair of long-sleeved disposable plastic gloves and a bottle of robust lubricant." Thank heavens, I thought, for generous men who helped elevate the status of women to full partnership in the profession or I might not be contemplating veterinary school at all.

Dr. Trout didn't think that a woman's size or sex had anything to do with her ability to control a hot-blooded stallion compared to the extra size of a male veterinarian. What could the extra 70 pounds matter, he reasoned, when faced with a ton of bridling equine. And he doubted that smaller salaries for vets, as claimed by males as a result of women entering the field, were a legitimate complaint because veterinarians were never as highly compensated as medical doctors; you just had to love your work. Vets didn't enter the practice to get rich. I liked that.

Along with other prospective veterinarians, I was allowed to sit in on the afternoon office hours in the veterinarian wing on campus. It was an opportunity to test out veterinary medicine, to see if we were truly interested. We were stationed behind one-way glass above the examining room. Dogs and their owners couldn't see us but we could see them.

Today a middle-aged, diminutive woman named Helen Piccard entered the examining room holding her German Shepherd, a beautiful animal, on a leash. It had a shiny fluffy coat, a full ruff around the neck, and was obviously well cared for and much beloved by his owner.

"Scooter's got some kind of growth at the back of his throat," said Mrs. Piccard, who was tugging on Scooter's leash with all the strength in her body. "You can see it, doctor, when you look down deep into his throat."

Dr. Hanley, the veterinarian, approached the dog, holding out his hand in a friendly manner; then he engagingly called the dog's name. Scooter, on his part, let out a low, menacing growl and the hair on his back rose.

"Oh, he's really just a pussycat," declared Mrs. Piccard. "It just takes him a moment to get acquainted."

That moment didn't arrive.

Dr. Hanley took the dog's collar and attempted to hold Scooter still so he could look into his mouth. But the dog let out another ominous growl, and the veterinarian thought better of his attempt and let the collar loose.

"How on earth did you discover the growth?" Dr. Hanley asked. "Scooter doesn't mind you peering down his throat?"

Mrs. Piccard answered in a voice indicating disapproval of Dr. Hanley's technique. "Why, my husband can peer down his throat any time he wants. He feeds him peanut butter, puts it right on his nose. When Scooter goes crazy trying to lick it off, you can see clear to the back of his throat."

13

Those of us observing couldn't suppress a laugh, picturing the dog's contortions as he tried to lick the peanut butter off his snout.

Dr. Hanley gamely continued the examination. "You haven't noticed blood dripping from his nose, Mrs. Piccard? Or around his bed? He's up to date on his shots?"

The woman nodded firmly.

"He continues to play with his toys? I remember he had a special ball."

"You'll lose a finger if you try to get one away from him," she said.

Dr. Hanley moved back a step in the interest of safety.

To our amusement, Dr. Hanley actually got down on the floor trying to see into Scooter's mouth, maintaining three feet of distance between their heads. I was afraid that Scooter might take it into his mind to bite off Dr. Hanley's nose.

Finally Dr. Hanley arose. "I'll be right back," he said. Minutes later he returned with a can of cat food, a wooden tongue depressor, and industrial-strength gloves. While we watched, he opened the can of cat food and placed a glob at the end of Scooter's nose, peanut butter style; then he waited for the dog to lift his tongue to lick it. When it did, Dr. Hanley quickly reached with his gloved fingers into the dog's mouth and peered inside. Finally he looked up, triumphant. "I see it," he exclaimed, "There it is; it's dime-sized. It'll definitely need to be biopsied. Mrs. Piccard, please hold his mouth shut while I feel his nymph nodes."

She looked anxiously at Dr. Hanley. "You'll be gentle with him, won't you, doctor? You know, he really is a pussycat."

"Of course he is," Dr. Hanley answered, trying to sound convincing.

Minutes later, as Mrs. Piccard and her pussycat departed, Dr. Hanley looked up at us through the window. "Next time he'll be anaesthetized," he grinned. "I advise you all to keep a can of cat food handy."

I made a note of it. It was an instructive class, and showed just how ingenious a veterinarian has to be.

CHAPTER THREE

I told my father about the program at the university. "They've got some good vets on their faculty," I said. "Many were trained at Angell Memorial Animal Center in Boston. They're tops in veterinary medicine."

Dad nodded. He'd been up all night delivering a baby and looked exhausted. He's 54 and his reddish hair is turning grey at his ears, but he's a good-looking man. "I already know about it, Amy. When I took my medical training at Harvard, I knew about Angell. Anyone who knows about veterinary medicine knows about Angell."

Then I told Dad about the veterinarian, Dr. Hanley, who put cat food on the dog's nose to distract it so he could see the growth at the back of his throat. "Very innovative," he said, laughing. "Vets have to learn some weird medical techniques just as we medical doctors do."

He hesitated and looked at me seriously. "You're doing all right, Amy?" he asked. "No more episodes? You look marvelous to me, darling. But you're a little thin."

I know he's worried about my bulimia, of course. I shook my head. "I'm all right, Dad. I hear that there's a support group at the university if I have trouble. I might look in on it."

"Good idea. Another thing—have you thought about working for a veterinary clinic this summer? I worked in a hospital during a vacation to see if I liked medicine and found that I did."

I cocked my head to one side, thinking about it. "It's a great idea, but where would I find a veterinary clinic willing to hire me?"

"I'll ask around. Most of my colleagues have animals. I'll find out if they can recommend one."

The more I thought about Dad's suggestion, the better I liked it. I didn't really know if I wanted to spend my entire life treating sick animals. The only experience I'd had was with Molly and with that veterinary class. The time to find out was now.

Mom's a sensible, bright woman, and I knew she'd probably bring eight more books home from the library about veterinary medicine, in addition to the ones I'd already read, if she thought I was serious about becoming a vet. We have books stacked under our dining room table so we can be prepared for anything we might discuss at dinner. That's the way it is when you have a mother who works at a library and a father who is eternally asking questions about science, history…or anything else. His curiosity is endless. When I had an astronomy project in high school, our topic for dinner the entire next week was the Milky Way. We had to look it up in the encyclopedia, discuss it, study it, and of course Mom brought home books about it from the library. By the time I handed the report in, I hoped I never had to look skyward again, but I got the best mark in the class.

Mom and Dad met in college, and when he went on to medical school, she took a graduate degree in library science. They married during Dad's senior year in medical school and eventually came to Centerville to live. Dad had grown up in Centerville and his parents, my grandparents, still live here, although they spend some of the year traveling to visit relatives. I was born and raised in Centerville and like being a small-town girl.

"I think your father is right about working in a clinic, sweetie," Mom said, concurring with my dad. "He mentioned it to me, too. Getting hands-on experience with a practicing veterinarian makes sense. Do you like the idea?"

"Sort of. It scares me a little. What if I'm not good enough and they tell me I can't do it?"

Mom put her arm around my shoulders. "You're good at what you do, Amy. I know you can do it if that's what you want to do."

My parents have faith in me, and I'll do all right if I don't beat myself up and tell myself that I'm a loser. I just can't fall into that rut again and start upchucking my meals. At least I know now that I was sick and that knowledge might carry me through. I also know that my parents are on tenterhooks thinking that they might say or do something to set me off again. But it doesn't work that way—it comes from inside me and maybe I've got it under control.

Dad actually does tell me the name of a clinic nearby, Veterinary Associates, where one of the surgeons takes his prize Samoyeds. I figure it must be an awfully good vet clinic to take care of such special dogs. Dad hands me the name of the clinic, its vet, Dr. Avery McDonald, and even the telephone number. So I screw up my courage and call them. I figure that Dad's colleague must have put in a good word for me so that I'm just not calling out of the blue.

A nice-sounding woman answers the phone. "You're Amy Richards?" she asks. "Dr. Mitchell mentioned you to Dr. McDonald, our head veterinarian. He said that you could drop by any afternoon at your convenience. Mornings here are for surgery."

"Great. Thanks. I'll come by tomorrow afternoon."

So the next day, there I am, at 3:30 in the afternoon. The clinic is a small building with dog pens in back, and, in front, a spacious, comfortable waiting room. The facade of the building is a tall arch, very imposing, with a door leading directly into the waiting room. A side door opens into a parking area. A statue of a large dog stands in the front yard, greeting everyone who enters.

Inside the building is a long counter in the center of the waiting room on which stands computers, paper forms, pens and pencils, and is presided over by three very busy women. One seems to be on the telephone nonstop, one is talking to patients paying bills, and a third signs out animals for release after they've been treated. It's a bustling place. A couple of wire dog pens stand in the corner, perhaps for animals who might need them while waiting for the doctor, or for those boarding here. In addition to the women at the desk is another talking to a man with a sick poodle who insists that his dog needs surgery now, right now, and that he's sorry he's four hours late. A woman, also awaiting the veterinarian, tugs a Beagle on a leash, saying it somehow opened her refrigerator door and ate almost the entire contents, including a loaf of bread, a pound of sliced turkey and another pound of cheese. "I think his tummy hurts," the woman adds tearfully. "See how big it is."

The poor dog's stomach looks like he'd swallowed a bowling ball, and the receptionist says she'll speak to the vet right away, to please wait. Just then a woman arrives with a drooping cat in a cage. The waiting room is filling rapidly with urgently sick animals.

As I wait to speak to one of the harassed women behind the desk, I read signs on the wall to pass the time. There's a whole wall devoted to lost pets. "Please return our Doberman," one sad sign pleads. "Its owner is despondent and very ill. He needs his Max." It was heartbreaking. Another says, "Sit, Stay. The doctor will be with you in a moment." It's a takeoff on the obedience command owners use to train their young pets, only this time it's directed toward pet owners. A wall hanging reads, "The pharaohs in ancient Greece considered cats to be gods, and cats have not forgotten this." I love it, knowing that someone around here has a sense of humor. Beyond the three women at the desk are two employees in coveralls moving in the rear offices, where I can see rooms with examining tables and an office. That's where the action is, I guess, where surgery is performed.

In fact, a man in green scrubs emerges from that office, confers with one of the women behind the counter, who waves a pen in my general direction. The man opens a little gate leading from the waiting room into that inner sanctum where a middle-aged man sits behind a large desk. He's also dressed in green coveralls, is of medium height with pepper and salt hair, and a tanned face. He has an air of authority. A stethoscope dangles about his neck and several tongue depressors peek from his breast pocket. I wonder if he has a can of cat food somewhere around here for dogs with growths in their throats.

"Hi, you must be Amy," he says, rising from the swivel chair behind the desk and extending his hand. His voice is kind. "I'm Dr. McDonald. Nice to meet you. I'm director of this clinic, or trying to be."

His office has pictures on all walls, mainly of dogs and cats but here and there is an occasional bird. Owners of those animals have written on the pictures testimonials to their happiness with the clinic's care of their pets. Books are stacked on a table, Dr. McDonald's desk, and on the floor. The place looks about like my college room at exam time, with books and stuff piled all over the place.

He indicates a chair opposite his desk, then sits down again in the swivel chair behind the desk. "Sorry about this place, but we've had a tough day around here. We're trying hard to catch up but it obviously isn't working. More surgery into the evening hours, I'm afraid."

He smiles over at me, then taps his pen on the desk pad and takes a breath. " I understand that you'd like to get some practical experience in a veterinary clinic. Is that right?"

I'm a little intimidated by this bustling place, but I manage to get my voice under control. "Yes, sir."

"I take it you've had no prior experience working with animals?"

What was I doing applying to this place, anyway? I'm almost embarrassed to confess my lack of experience. "I have a dog. But I'd be glad to help out any way I can during the summer. If you need help, I mean, I can learn." I'm thinking, I like this clinic. I'd like to work here.

"Well, I understand that you're very bright, Amy. I know your father a little and he's a good man."

"Yes, sir, he is."

"And as you can see, we need help. Although every day isn't this bad."

I nod knowingly, having seen the chaos in the outer office.

"And you understand that we couldn't pay very much."

"Well, I didn't expect…"

"We could use someone to sweep the floor around here after patients—two-footed and four-footed—have gone for the day. And to feed the animals we keep overnight. Someone comes in to monitor them then so that wouldn't be your responsibility. To help clean out cages now and then and assist with grooming; We have a small but loyal clientele. If things work out, perhaps you could even help in the examining rooms." A smile flickers across his face. "Not very glamorous, is it? But that's what goes on in a vet's office. Excepting surgery, of course. We handle some pretty bizarre cases sometimes."

I was tempted to tell him about the dog with cat food on his nose but decided that this man was too harassed for stories. "I'd like to try, Dr. McDonald. If you think I can help…I'll do my best." If it didn't sound glamorous, it was what I wanted, and I had to start somewhere. Actually, I was pretty relieved that he would even consider me.

"When could you start?"

"In a month. That's when school lets out.'

"All right. That'll be when some of my staff goes on vacation so I think we can fit you in. You're not afraid of snakes, are you? Or hamsters? Gerbils?"

I take a short breath. "Snakes…a little. I had hamsters when I was little. My brother owned gerbils. One is still lost in a wall of our house."

Dr. McDonald laughs. "We'll keep you on dogs. Don't worry, you'll get used to our patients."

I shake hands again with Dr. McDonald and leave. I know I was smiling.

I call Ruth, who is also at home on school break. I think my voice is squeaking. "I got the job, Ruth. Can you believe it?"

"You mean it? That's great, kiddo. Yes, I can believe it. Now if I can just land one at my mother's hospital…"

"You will, I know you will. I can feel it in my bones."

"I hope that your bones are psychic." She hesitated. "You're feeling okay?"

She knew that a crisis could set me off again, but this was not a crisis; it was a triumph. "I'm fine, Ruth. Don't worry." I get the weird feeling that every one who knew about my bulimia would worry about me forever. It's very uncomfortable, but I appreciate their concern just the same.

"When is your interview?" I ask Ruth. "Soon, I hope. We don't have much spring break left."

Ruth laughs. "Mom says I really don't need an interview because they're always short of help. They'll take me on my mother's recommendation. Besides, half the staff knows me already because I've visited the hospital often enough to see my Mom."

"That's great."

Ruth nods. "You know how lucky we are to get jobs? Health is the only field hiring, Mom says. Say, do you want to celebrate tonight? We could try The Pub on Main Street. They have pizza, and some of the college crowd already hangs out there."

I'm in the mood. "Can you get a car, or do you want me to ask Mom?"

"She already said I could take hers. I'll pick you up around six."

Neither of us had taken time off during the vacation. I'd had a paper to finish for comparative anatomy, and Ruth was completing a project for psychology. "I need some fun before heading back to school," Ruth says.

"All work and no play…" I echo.

The Pub is really a beer joint but it also serves food the college crowd can afford. It's a short distance from the center of town near a small grocery store, a discount hardware, and a furniture factory. We already know most of the college kids, because they've been in our high school classes, and now a couple even live in our dorms at the university. Five or six from other colleges are also home on vacation, about to return just as we are. "Hey, Ruthy," a stringy beanpole of a guy calls out and waves as we enter the place. It has a bar along one wall and a mirror above it, like in old western movies, and the place smells of cheese and fried onions. "Come over and join the crowd," calls the beanpole. The "crowd" is holding forth at several tables, which had been shoved together in the middle of the room.

"Hey, Mike," Ruth answers, waving. I follow her over to join the others. Ruth is pretty popular and the guys as well as the girls like her. We greet everyone and sit down at the first table next to Mike.

A girl at my elbow says, "How'ya doing, Amy? Having a good vacation?" She was in my comparative anatomy class at the university, but I'd sat next to her in high school chemistry.

I beam. "Just got a summer job, Terri. I'm pretty happy about it."

"No kidding. Where? I've been looking."

"In a veterinary office."

"You're going to vet school? But isn't that awfully hard training? Don't you have to take extra years for a degree?"

"Sure, but it doesn't take as long as achieving a degree for either a medical doctor or veterinarian at another university because it's a combined degree. What are you planning to do? This summer, I mean?"

"Work for my father, I guess. He's an accountant. I think I'll go to summer school to learn the ropes."

"Good for you."

Another guy, Rod Towns, shows up behind us. He's tall, very good looking, and knows it. He was in my lit class. "You're planning to be a vet, Amy? You don't mean it? You wanna go broke? Vets don't make much money, you know."

"I don't intend to make lots of money, Rod. That's not why I'm thinking of being a vet. I like animals. I'm going to try a course or two to see if I like it."

He makes a face. "Can't imagine. I'm heading to law school."

He's an arrogant snob and I don't want to talk to him, but somehow he's sitting beside me. "Good for you," I manage in a cool voice.

But he's leaning over me. "My cousin just had my dog put to sleep. Ugh! You want to kill animals?"

"I don't intend to kill animals, Rod. I want to help them."

"Well, I intend to help people and make money."

Ruth turns back, having been talking to someone beside her. "You'll make a fine lawyer," she jokes. "Do you intend to buy a bank to hold all your money?"

He stops with a cold look on his face. "What's that supposed to mean?" he asks Ruth. "Something wrong with lawyers?"

"Of course not. I was just joking."

I get my back up. "She wants to be a nurse. You don't approve of that, either?" I respond, bristling. "It takes a lot of skill to be a nurse as well as a veterinarian. I don't know about lawyers. I'm beginning to wonder."

He pauses a minute, backing off. "Like I said, you're not going where the big money is."

"Making 'big money' isn't for everyone."

He looks at Ruth, then at me, and turns away, obviously wanting to hang out with more enlightened types. "I'm glad you challenged him," Ruth says. "He's in my history class. Not many people can stand him."

"Well, he's right about one thing. I can't imagine putting a dog to sleep. It gives me nightmares."

"Maybe you won't have to," Ruth answers. "Don't listen to people like him. He's a joke."

"I know. But for a moment there, I got a sinking feeling."

She glances at me, scrutinizing my face.

I catch her glance. "Don't worry, Ruth. I'm really okay. I'm fine "

"I'm not worrying, Amy. I just don't want guys like that putting you down."

"I can handle it." For the first time I actually feel that maybe I can.

I've got two more days of vacation and then back to school. Ruth and I ride back to the university with Ruth's mom. My mother had picked us up two weeks ago. We're feeling lucky because we both have jobs. It seems a sort of miracle.

I'm looking forward to getting back to the university. In fact, I can't wait.

CHAPTER FOUR

In my classes, I continue to get good marks. Some of us who are interested in becoming veterinarians are allowed to return frequently to the viewing window in the veterinary college examining room, usually on Thursday afternoons. It's an amazing and instructive look into veterinary medicine. I love it because I can see and hear, through sound piped into the room, how veterinarians work and how they diagnose animals' problems.

Some dog owners, I find, dote on their animals and hover over the vet to make sure he doesn't handle them roughly. The vets I saw showed great care for the animals they handled and made every effort to understand how sensitive little Poopsy is. I realize that if I become a vet, I'll have to get used to the quirky concerns of pet owners, but most love their dogs dearly. One woman came in during one session in front of the viewing window with a small dog, a Chihuahua, dressed in a pink sweater and matching skirt extending out from its tiny fanny. It looked like a circus dog imitating a ballerina. The owner baby talked to the animal, kissed it on its nose, and fluttered over it like a mother with a newborn.

"You know," she told Dr. Selkirk, the vet in the examining room that day, "dog mouths are much cleaner than human mouths. I have to brush my teeth before I kiss Poopsy. You can't be too sure you won't pass on nasty human germs to innocent dogs."

Amazingly to me, the vet agreed. "Dog's kisses are quite harmless compared to those of humans," he said, "unless we're talking about rabies, a disease which affects dogs and people in equally damaging ways. But humans are generally immune to most dog diseases. Likewise, most human germs don't affect dogs. But a bite from a human mouth full of harmful bacteria may well be more damaging than a dog bite."

The woman continued with her display of dog knowledge: "A dog's kiss has healing power because the strong enzymes in the saliva are cleansing and curative."

"It all depends," interrupted Dr. Selkirk, "on what the human and dog have put in their mouths lately. Humans don't tend to chew on dead animals or get into garbage the way dogs do. Frankly, I'd rather have a French kiss with a human than a dog."

We all laughed, though the woman looked unconvinced.

Another observation I made at the window was how often dogs resemble their owners. Small, feminine women seemed to own small dogs, which many carry around in pouches. They tie bows in their hair and spray their coats with perfume and speak lisping talk to them. Setters belonged to athletic men or women who take long walks with their pets, wrestle with them, or include them in boating and hunting trips. During one observation period, an overweight bulldog with heavy jowls belonging to a big, overweight man with equally heavy jowls, seemed to dare the vet to get him onto the examining table. The dog, Bruno, didn't budge when the vet tugged on his leash and tried to coax the animal near the table. Bruno seemed stuck to the floor.

"Bruno jes don't like bein' handled," confided the owner. "He's pretty partic'lar."

The vet surveyed the situation. "So am I. You get him near the table and I'll help get him on board."

The owner attempted to throw a lock hold onto Bruno's hind section, but Bruno swished his rear and managed to elude his owner's efforts. Finally, with the combined exertions of the vet and the owner, they managed to hoist the corpulent animal onto the examining table so that the vet could proceed with his examination. Finally, still winded, the vet rendered his verdict: "This animal needs to be on a diet," he declared emphatically. "It wouldn't hurt him a bit to lose 50 pounds."

Those of us in the viewing window again went into gales of laughter, because it was so obvious that the owner needed to be put on a diet, too.

Setters seemed to belong to outdoor people who often ran with them; Chihuahuas to feminine women who treated them like dolls, often providing them with a full wardrobe of clothing matching the raiments of the owner. One woman told the veterinarian that she read her dog stories before it went to bed at night. Although such behavior was tender and kind, it was so bizarre that I thought some dogs were a little crazy because their owners were, too.

Another woman and man, owners of a beloved Great Pyrenees dog, gave the animal a birthday party every year to which they invited all the dogs in the neighborhood, serving gourmet meats and dog treats. The couple, obviously used to things on a generous scale—including their homes, possessions, and influence in their world—treated the fortunate dog to the same pampered lifestyle.

I completed the first semester with an A average. My dad was impressed. "I told you that you could go into anything you want," he said. "You'll do well at whatever you try, Amy."

I realized that he was still subtly pushing medical school again, sort of giving me a second chance to change my mind. "Dad, I really like what I've seen of veterinary medicine. It fascinates me. I'd like to go on with it. I'll love saving animals' lives."

"But you're saving real lives when you treat human beings."

"But people depend on their dogs. Sometimes their dogs save lives, as Molly saved mine. Seeing Eye dogs guide thousands of people who couldn't survive without them, but ordinary mutts provide companionship for shut-ins in nursing homes and hospitals. Sometimes dogs seem like people to their owners, giving comfort, loyalty, and even protection to them."

We were in my father's study, an inner sanctum where the walls are lined with medical books, and where my father retreats to read medical journals. His face was serious, his forehead furrowed with fatigue. I definitely didn't want to follow in his footsteps. I respected and loved him but I felt sorry for him.

"I want what you want, Amy, but please think about the future. "It's coming up awfully fast, and this is the time to make plans."

"I know, Dad. I'm giving it my attention." He was thinking about my brother who really wanted to follow my father into medicine, and making a last try for me to consider his field. I'd known that fact all during my teenage years, and felt that in some way I was betraying a wish. I'd lived in my brother's shadow for years, and I loved that. I did it willingly, with happiness and joy. But I also knew that I couldn't follow in my brother's path—my brother wasn't here and I was. Besides, my health was still precarious. I couldn't live my brother's life, much as I adored him. And much as I loved my father, I had to go my way.

I talked to Mom about it. It was after dinner and we'd taken a walk, with Molly trailing behind. I'd stopped to pet her, feeling her silky coat. I was proud of her and eternally thankful to my grandparents for letting her stay with me during vacations. She kept me company and had become my stalwart companion. I talked to her all the time, and I know that she understood most of what I had to say. Sometimes I swear that she talked back with her expressions. Other times she'd lick my hand or bark happily or wag her silky tail.

"Dad means well and loves you dearly, darling. He wants what you want for yourself and agrees wholeheartedly. But he's still brokenhearted about Brian." Mom pushed a wisp of hair from her forehead. Mom, a dark blond, is turning faintly gray. "Give him time. Sometimes we just have to stand up for ourselves. It isn't easy but we all have to do it. Who knows, maybe Brian wouldn't have wanted to go into medicine. Besides, being a veterinarian is medicine, too, and I understand it's very difficult. Your father wouldn't have a clue how to treat a dog, or cat, hamster, or snake. Can you really treat a snake with a sore throat? I mean, how do you get a light down...?"

We started to laugh, trying to picture Dad peering down a snake's throat, and it restored my confidence. My mom has always had a way to make me feel better.

Two days later, I returned to the university from spring break. Ruth said, "How did it go, Amy? Is your Dad still hoping you'll forget about veterinary school?"

"Yes, but he won't push very hard. I know my Dad and he'll get used to it."

"I know he will, Amy. He's still grieving about Brian."

I nodded. "If Brian had lived, I think he'd have gone into practice with Dad. It was Dad's dream."

We had gone to the cafeteria for a quick lunch and my free time was fleeting until the next class, a seminar. "I agree with what your Mom said, Amy, that maybe he wouldn't have gone into medicine. Who knows?"

I nodded. Who did know?

"Listen, hang in there, girl," Ruth said. She'd cut her hair during vacation and I loved the way her blond hair curled about her face. "Don't give up. Hey, maybe I can help you out sometime when I get my nursing degree. Except I wouldn't know what to do with a sick frog."

We both laughed. "Neither would I, Ruth. Luckily, the clinic mostly limits its practice to dogs and cats. Although Dr. McDonald asked me how I felt about handling gerbils and hamsters and snakes."

"Snakes? Wasn't he kidding?"

"I hope so. I told him I preferred gerbils and hamsters."

"How does one operate on a hamster or snake?"

I laughed again. "I don't know but I'll tell you when I find out."

"Agreed. By the way, I ran into your buddy, Rod Towns, the other day. The guy we met at The Pub, going into law school?"

I picked up my books from the table. "He's not my buddy, Ruth."

"I know. I'm just kidding. Well, he asked about you."

"About me? Why was he asking about me?"

She smiled. "You know, I think he likes you a little."

"Ruth, Rod thinks I'm an idiot for even thinking of going to vet school. I think he's an idiot for planning to go to law school. He's a jerk. Lawyers sue doctors."

"I'm just telling you what he said. He thinks you're very pretty."

That stopped me cold. "Pretty? He said that? That proves he's an idiot." I'd touched up my dark hair with red highlights when Mom had hers colored. I'd always considered my hair mousy and I'd never thought of myself as pretty. But my hair did look nice.

"You *are* pretty, Amy. That's what I keep telling you. Why don't you believe me?"

That's what Mom kept telling me. "'You're an attractive girl, Amy, and a wonderful daughter. I wish I could convince you.'"

I've been told that when you have bulimia, it's partly because you have a poor mental image of yourself. I couldn't help it. But I felt a lift from Ruth's words. It was actually the first time I'd considered the

29

possibility that I was good-looking. I'd have to go home and look at myself in the mirror. I gave her a hug. "How's nursing going, Ruth?" I asked. "You're still enthusiastic?"

"I love it. Mom and I talk about it all the time. Even my father is pleased, and he's an engineer. Half the time he doesn't even know what we're talking about. Hospital jargon sounds like Greek to him."

We laughed at that, but just the same, I wish I had that bond with my father, the way Ruth shares her profession with her Mom. Yet I know they love me and that Dad will eventually understand that I've chosen my field and won't change my mind. I think he even admires me for it.

I waved goodbye to Ruth, refreshed by lunch and her company, and we headed back to our afternoon classes.

CHAPTER FIVE

I'd spoken to a couple of veterinarians at the vet school about the difficulty of entering their program, and one even took time to look at my grades. Afterward, he really encouraged me. I'd actually seen him before through that viewing window; it was Dr. Hanley. "Have you needed to put cat food on a dog's nose lately?" I asked him. I couldn't hide a smile.

"You saw that?" He groaned. "I'm still trying to live it down with my colleagues. But I notice that now there are cans of cat food in the medical closet."

"And you succeeded in finding the dog's growth in his throat. We were all impressed."

"Thanks." He laughed. "Good luck on your studies, Amy. I'm glad you're interested in veterinary medicine. Come to see me if you want to chat about it anytime."

He was very nice. Up close, he was probably several years older than me, nice looking, with a full head of wavy brown hair. Like my Dad, he carried his stethoscope around his neck. And because he was an instructor in the school, I figured that he must be pretty smart. I knew by now that getting into vet school was more difficult than being

31

chosen for med school, so this man must be the brightest of the bright. I'd have to ace my studies to make the grade.

Doubts overtook me just thinking about it, but at least I could try. If I didn't try, I'd for sure not make it. That was frightening to me, but just by making the effort, I had hope in my life. I could think about the future without panicking or wanting to binge and purge like all bulimics, and maybe the next decision would come easier. Please, God, I thought, I really want to do this.

I reported to the veterinary clinic the day after I started summer vacation. The semester had dragged on so long that I was afraid they might have given the job to someone else by now. I'd called a month ago, worried they'd forgotten all about me, so they'd know I was still alive and eager. I didn't trust their memories one bit to recall, in their frantic schedule, a single interview with a lone applicant six weeks ago.

I walked into the clinic with my stomach clenched tight because I wasn't sure I could handle the work they wanted me to do, even if it was menial. Menial was relative when you hadn't done it before—to me it was going to be a mighty effort just to learn new procedures.

I spoke to a red-haired woman sitting behind the counter who I recalled from my first visit here to apply for a job. She remembered me and told me that Dr. McDonald was in surgery, but that a woman in the back office named Grace would show me around. Grace arrived almost immediately with a smile and a welcoming handshake. She was middle-aged, tall, strong and competent-looking. "Welcome aboard," she said. "We're a little short-handed right now, so Dr. McDonald said to put you to work right away." I wouldn't even have time to be nervous!

In the clinic there were three vets, I discovered, as well as the three women I'd seen in the outer office to handle the patient load, and four or five workers to help with various aspects of the practice. Along with Dr. McDonald, one of the other vets, Dr. Stokes, was in surgery when I arrived and Dr. Dubin was on a conference call.

So Grace showed me the ropes. I would help keep the dog food stocked, maintain cleanliness in the outside pens, assist the groomers when requested, and help the vets in the examining room. This would really be a busy, hands-on apprenticeship.

Grace took me into a back storeroom to point out the animal food, and to indicate the portions allotted to the animals being boarded over night. She pointed out, in an isolation area reserved for contagious animals, a small dog in a cage with a disease named parvovirus which, she indicated, was often a killer among young dogs like this one. The poor thing was absolutely limp, with no desire to eat, so they were feeding the little dog intravenously with a tube in his leg. His ears drooped, he was emaciated, and couldn't lift his head. When Grace opened his cage to check him, she said I could pet him. I rubbed him gently behind the ears but he never moved. Grace told me to put on rubber gloves and to change the soiled bedding under the little fellow two or three time a day.

In the next cage was a kitten abandoned by its mother, being fed milk from a baby bottle. I held the bottle while it licked the nipple. At least, Grace said, he was getting stronger and would be weaned in a day or two.

In other cages Grace introduced dogs recovering from surgery. One, an English lab named Morgan, had swallowed its leash. How could a dog swallow its leash, I wondered. Why would it swallow a leash? I was soon to discover that animals swallow all manner of foreign substances, which subsequently need removal. It had already undergone three operations to remove the leash and to plug the perforations in its stomach and bowel. The dog was obviously in pain and its prognosis was not optimistic. The owner, a schoolteacher, told Grace he couldn't afford more surgeries.

But then an odd thing happened. In the waiting room, while the schoolteacher and his wife are holding hands and crying, a burly construction worker entered with his mastiff.

"What's the trouble?" he asked the stricken couple. When they explained how sick their dog had become as the result of swallowing the leash, and that they were going to have to put Morgan down, the worker placed his massive hand on the schoolteacher's shoulder. "There, there," he said, patting the man's shoulder as if soothing a child, "You jes' can't put a nice dog like that down. You love 'im. Why don't you give him one more surgery before you let him go."

Grace broke into a big smile. "Well, wouldn't you know, the couple perked up, Dr. Stokes and Dr. McDonald operated one more time, and that dog is going to make it. It's beyond belief."

She pointed proudly to the cage where Morgan, a thin but handsome dog, was devouring the food we'd just put in his bowl. "You keep it up," Grace told the dog, "and you'll be going home in no time. Just don't swallow any more leashes." I was as proud of that dog as Grace was, and I'd had nothing to do with saving him. But now he would be part of my responsibility.

I noticed that several of the cages had toys in them. Therein was another story from Grace. "Our clients continually bring in favorite toys for their dogs," she said. "You'll find blankets in the cages, and monogrammed sweaters in case their dog gets chilled, and balls, even though the animals are too sick to play. Most owners bring dog dishes from home, or pick them up at Walmart; but other dogs arrive at the clinic with fancy china including their animal's name on the bowl."

Grace told me of a woman who brought her dog into the clinic with a bottle of perfume, saying that little Bitsie couldn't fall asleep without a dab behind her ears and on her paws before she went to sleep. "Course," Grace told me confidentially, "the dog slept perfectly well when we forgot to give her perfume, but I'm not about to tell the owner."

Grace had a treasure trove of stories about clinic clients "One dog," she went on, "arrived with two goose-down pillows with the price tag still attached. They were $199 each. Another client who calls her dogs 'kids,' brought in a gadget like a pinball machine with a handle shaped like a bone that the 'kids' could press to get a doggie snack. The owner also bought her dogs matching leather bomber jackets with lambskin collars costing $300 each. She told the staff that she couldn't take her money with her so what better way to spend it than to lavish it on her animals?"

I gasped. "Was she a little crazy?"

"Not as nuts as the woman with a neurotic dog who sent the animal to Denmark for private psychiatric therapy. She chartered a private jet and stayed in a four-star hotel for a month. When asked about it, she told Dr. McDonald that it was only $5,000 more expensive than she'd anticipated."

I could have listened to Grace all day. A veterinary practice was unlike anything I'd heard of before. At least the owners were devoted to their dogs, and if their devotion was excessive, it was also heartwarming. I overheard one client telling Dr. McDonald that her dog had stopped chewing slippers, socks, pillows, and upholstery when he discovered

Animal Planet. The dog would sit on the couch attentively watching television when the owner left the house on an errand, and nothing would have been destroyed during her absence. Another was addicted to soap operas. That owner apparently said to Dr. Stokes, much to his amusement, "My dog has taste in his arse." Dogs seemed to have as many quirks as humans.

That night Ruth and I compared notes over burgers at The Pub. "They're giving me lots more responsibility than I expected," Ruth said, smothering her hamburger under gobs of ketchup. "They're so short-handed that they don't have time to carry supplies from one area to the other. I'm taking temperatures, blood pressures, and monitoring medications. I'm on the same ward as my Mom, so I get a chance to look over her shoulder."

I laughed. "I'm feeding dogs and cats," I told her. Then I related the story Grace had told me about the dog who swallowed its leash. "He's getting better day by day. He's thin as a rail, but…"

Just then I caught sight of Rod Towns entering the restaurant with a girl. I didn't look up but told Ruth quietly. "Don't look now, but our favorite budding attorney just arrived."

"Terrific," she said. "But I don't think he'll be as rude to you as he was last time."

I made a face. "You think he's had a sudden change of heart?"

"Maybe. I gave him a piece of my mind when I ran into him on campus after spring break. He may have thought twice about it afterward."

"I doubt it. But thanks, Ruth."

To my surprise, he left his table and came over to ours. "Hi, there," he said to both of us. "Are you both having a good summer?"

I nodded, not about to elaborate.

Ruth looked at him. "You're working in your Dad's law office, Rod?"

"Yep. It isn't half bad." He turned to me. "I hear you're working for a vet, Amy."

I barely looked at him. "Three of them, actually." I actually smirked. "It isn't half bad, either." I couldn't resist the words coming out with a sarcastic edge.

His face actually softened a little. "Listen, Amy, I'm sorry if I was rude the other day. Ruth let me have it."

"You bet I did," Ruth agreed. "You deserved it."

"I agree," he said. " I was pissed off about something and took it out on you."

"I pissed you off?" I asked. "I don't even know you."

He shook his head. "I got a bad mark in one of my classes. My Dad was furious about it, said I'd never make law school with my attitude. I know he was right but it rubbed me the wrong way."

Ruth and I were quiet, evaluating his apology. Then Ruth smiled. "Just don't let it happen again. Amy and I aren't used to snide remarks."

He nodded. "Agreed."

I looked over at him. "Thanks for apologizing."

"Well, I'll see you around," he said, looking at each of us. Then with a little wave, he turned back to his date.

"Miracles never cease," Ruth said after he'd gone. "Maybe he isn't such a bad guy, after all."

"Let's hope," I answered. "But I don't want to put him to the test."

CHAPTER SIX

One Saturday morning a week later, I was vacuuming my bedroom, a much overdue effort, while Molly sat on my bed, cocking her head from side to side as she watched the unfamiliar activity. Then the phone rang on the extension on my desk. I turned off the vacuum and answered the phone.

"Hi," said a deep voice at the other end.

"Hi, Rod," I answered, not feeling like talking.

"Are you busy?" His voice actually sounded tentative, not full of the bluster I'd heard before.

"I'm cleaning house. What do you want?" If I sounded terribly abrupt, I didn't really care.

"Well, I just want to say hello, and to apologize again for being so rude the other day."

"Thank you. Apology accepted." You were rude, I thought.

"I mean, I shot my mouth off. I don't know any veterinarians, but I'm sure they're really...nice."

"But broke," I retorted. I felt like adding, not like rich lawyers, but I got hold of myself at the last minute.

"Listen, Amy, I just wanted to ask you if you wanted to go for a walk with me this afternoon. It's a really nice day. Then you can throw a rock at me if you feel like it."

I hesitated. "I really might, you know."

"Well, I deserve it. But I know a really nice trail in the woods. I'd like some company if you would."

I was about to tell him to forget it, that I had more important things to do. But when I looked around, sun was streaming in the window. It was a gorgeous day. I'd love to stop this idiotic cleaning and I hadn't walked all week. "If I can bring my dog," I said.

"Sure. Lots of people bring their dogs on the trail."

That decided it. Molly needed exercise, too.

"Would you be ready about 2?" he asked.

"Okay. Sure. We'll be ready. But no cracks about veterinarians. Molly gets offended easy."

He laughed. "I wouldn't dare. I promise."

I called Ruth. "You're not going to believe it, but Rod asked me to take a walk with him, Ruth. Is this crazy, or what? I even told him I'd go."

"That's great, Amy. I told you he said he was sorry."

"Well, we'll see about that."

"Call me when you get back, okay? He could turn out to be a nicer guy than we thought."

When I told my Mom what I was doing, she said, "I wouldn't tell your father if I were you, Amy. Mr. Towns is suing one of your Dad's colleagues. But it has nothing to do with you or his son." I actually think that my mother was pleased I was going out, and didn't give a second thought about what the men were scrapping about in their professions.

Rod arrived almost on the dot of 2:00. He actually smiled when he saw me. He was taller than I recalled, with light grey eyes, a rounded chin, dark hair covered by a Red Sox hat, and a tan which indicated that he'd been spending time outdoors. He was dressed in jeans, as I was, and wore a long-sleeved shirt under a sweatshirt with the school colors, blue and yellow. I'd found a pair of hiking shoes at the back of my closet, so I figured I was as ready as I could be for a trek into the woods with Rod Towns--unless I brought that rock.

"Thanks for coming," he said, sounding really sincere, as I stepped out onto my front walk. He didn't seem half as wiseass as at our last encounter. I introduced him to Molly, who was happily wagging her tail in anticipation of an outing. We climbed into Rod's car, a late-model Honda. I shoved Molly into the back seat along with Rod's stuff: notebooks, newspapers, a couple of sweaters and a volleyball.

"Sorry for the mess," he said, looking at me apologetically. "I'm having to repeat a course--math--at the junior college this summer. Those are workbooks. It's a real drag."

Obviously he was taking it hard that he had to repeat a subject, but maybe it had humbled him a little.

"Molly won't bother anything," I reassured Rod. "She loves to travel in a car. She'll just sit and look out the window at other cars." I looked back at her, and she had her nose out the window as the breeze ruffled her coat.

"You mean it? Don't most animals need to be restrained in cars?"

"Not Molly. She's very calm and obedient. She loves a little excitement." I looked over at him "Don't you have a dog or cat?"

He shook his head. "My mother's allergic to animal hair. We never had any pets. Not even fish." He laughed at the revelation.

So he didn't know a thing about animals. I felt a little sorry for him.

"How's it going at your clinic?" he asked.

"Great," I answered. "I like the work. The doctors are nice, too, and so is the staff. I'm learning a lot."

"Like what?" At first I thought that he was questioning what I could possibly learn in a veterinary clinic, but then I decided that wasn't it at all. He couldn't very well be gloating when he'd flunked a class. He just didn't know the first thing about veterinarians. Still, he seemed interested.

I looked at his profile as he drove the car. "It takes a lot of skill to diagnose what's wrong with an animal," I explained. "They can't tell you where it hurts."

He nodded and thought about it a minute as he was driving. "So how do you ever treat a sick animal?" he asked. "It sounds impossible to me."

CATHERINE A. HOSMER

"It takes expertise and ingenuity," I acknowledged. I again related the cat-food-on-the-nose story. "Sometimes you have to use your imagination."

He laughed at the picture of a vet on his hands and knees peering down a dog's throat. "I never could do that," he said. "I just don't connect that way with animals. Sometimes I wish I did because everyone else does." He looked into the rearview mirror. "Your Molly seems like a good dog."

I turned to see Molly contentedly thrusting her nose even farther out the open window, the ruff around her neck blowing in the breeze. "She *is* a good dog. She belongs to my grandparents, but she spends time with me when I'm home from school." I didn't want to tell him the circumstances which led to my having the dog so I changed the subject. "How's your summer going?" I asked him.

"Okay, I guess. I'm not working full time with my Dad until I get the course out of the way."

"How long do you have?"

"Four more weeks. I'm just not very good at math."

I'd always been good at math, but I wasn't about to tell him. "You need math to get into law school?"

"Big time. Sometimes lawyers must analyze really complicated financial statements. They have to be whizzes at math."

Sometimes I have trouble balancing my checkbook, so I wouldn't have a clue how to analyze a financial statement. Nor would I particularly want to. But I could see how flunking math could be a drawback to a lawyer.

The park was a short distance out of town. Rod eased the car into the parking area, alongside several other cars. It looked as if this was a popular destination on this nice Saturday afternoon. A few families were seated at the picnic tables enjoying a meal, and kids were playing on the swings and slides. I'd picnicked here with my parents when my brother was alive, but I hadn't been back since. I remember when Brian and Dad played softball with a group of men on the diamond nearby, but I quickly looked away, feeling the pain of that memory.

The trail Rod had chosen started with a climb, and then leveled off into a woods. Molly was beside herself sniffing with mounting excitement at all the ripe forest smells. Undoubtedly rabbits had crossed the path recently, leaving behind delectable scents irresistible to dogs.

40

And here and there she saw a squirrel, which led to a wild chase until Molly found that she couldn't climb a tree.

We hiked through a shaded pine grove, mottled with sunshine, where wildflowers like lupine, bluebells and forget-me-nots were already blooming. Apple blossoms from a few gnarled wild apple trees along the way sent a deliciously sweet smell into the air. Molly ran back and forth along the trail, then dove into the clear water of a small brook which joined us a short way into the trail. When she shook water over both of us, Rod didn't complain; in fact, he actually laughed at her antics.

"How did you ever find this trail?" I asked Rod. "I've been to the park but didn't know it was here. It's lovely."

"I've hiked it with my brother," he said. "He's in prep school, but he'll be home soon. He's two years younger than I am."

I felt immediately sad again. Was I going to be sad my entire life, thinking about Brian? "I...I had a brother, too," I said, and then could have bitten my tongue off for having volunteered that information.

Rod stopped on the trail ahead of me. "'Had?' What happened to him?"

I swallowed hard. "He was killed in the Iraq war."

He stared at me. "What a shame! Sorry, I didn't know."

"I'm trying to get over it, but I don't think I ever will."

He shook his head. "A couple of my buddies got killed in it, too. What a useless war."

"Well, it's still going on. My parents think we'll have soldiers over there for decades. They're trying to recover, too."

He picked up a stick from the ground and snapped it into pieces. "I wouldn't want to go. That's for sure."

"I wish my brother hadn't gone, but he was gung-ho, like a few other boys in his class. Dad tried to talk him out of it, Mom cried, but there was no pulling him back once he'd made his decision.

We continued, not talking. The trail ended on the top of a hill where we could see down into the valley and to the other side.

"It's nice up here," I told Rod finally as we looked down at roofs of farmhouses below us. Molly stood next to me, wondering what we were going to do next. I patted the top of her head and she licked my hand.

"My father's parents once lived down there," Rod said, looking out into the distance. "They had a small farm. My grandfather grew all the food they ate."

"Really? That's hard work!"

"It was, but my grandfather loved it. He was a born farmer. In his spare time, he did woodcarving. He carved dogs and horses…and even people. I still have a few of his pieces."

"They still live there?"

He shook his head. "They died in a flu epidemic a few years ago. The farm sold and a developer took over the land. He really confiscated the property, according to my father. I think that's why Dad decided to become a lawyer. He was outraged that his parents could be victimized that way, and that the guy could get away with it. In the meantime, I got interested in the law, too."

"I'm sure it's very interesting."

He smiled. "As long as it doesn't involve math."

We turned around and headed back, Molly trailing reluctantly at our heels. We met other hikers walking up the trail as we returned. We found Rod's car in the parking lot, Molly climbed into the back seat, and I settled myself in front.

"Thanks," I told Rod as he backed up the car. "I enjoyed the hike. I was feeling pretty housebound."

"You didn't feel the urge to throw a rock?"

I laughed. "Not once. You didn't make any cracks about veterinarians, either."

He smiled. "And Molly was a perfect lady."

"Of course. She saved my life."

"She did? How come?" He turned to look at me.

Now I'd let it out, and I didn't know how he'd take it. But what did I care? Yet I did, to my surprise. "Well, I was bulimic after Brian died. My grandparents loaned Molly to me, thinking she would help. Dogs are good companions for all kinds of problems and illnesses. Seeing Eye dogs save lives. Molly saved mine."

"You mean it?" He looked back at Molly, riding so happily in the back seat.

"She wouldn't let me out of her sight. I had to let her out, feed her and play with her. I think she restored my faith in life. I was about to give it up at one time."

He actually reached over for my hand. "You had a lot of courage," he said. I'm glad you made it."

I smiled. "So am I."

"I haven't related to people all that well myself, as you could tell by my bluster. I'm trying to reform." He smiled. "I know I'm improving …you didn't throw a rock."

I laughed. "I've got a secret: I wasn't about to…not even once." Maybe, I thought, everyone has hard times in their lives at one time or another

As we approached my home, I turned to Rod. "Thanks," I said. "I've enjoyed being with you today."

"We'll do it again," he promised.

Molly and I watched him disappear down the road. Then I called Ruth. "It was fun," I told her. "It surprised me. Even Molly had a good time."

"I'm glad, Amy. Mom says that Rod's father can be overbearing. He was in the hospital once and drove the nurses crazy. Maybe that explains why Rod can be so brusque sometimes."

"He says he's trying to reform."

"Well, I sure hope he succeeds."

"Maybe he will."

CHAPTER SEVEN

The veterinary clinic was bustling on Monday morning. Apparently a group of dogs, all purchased at a local mall, were sick and had been brought in by their owners for treatment. The owners were understandably upset. One of the young dogs had a broken leg, and several others were stricken with skin and bone diseases. All were malnourished and filthy.

"What's wrong with them?" I asked Grace. I'd been feeding them, and each one appeared sicker than the last. "They look miserable."

"I agree. They're in a deplorable state."

"Why would anyone have purchased one of these animals?"

Grace appeared as distraught as I was. "I wish I knew, Amy. I suppose it's because they're cheap. When kids see them at the mall, they fall in love with them. Then Mom buys one, takes it home, and finds it's sick."

"But where do they come from?"

"I suspect that someone's got a puppy mill not far away," she explains. "We're seeing more and more of these poor animals every day."

"A 'puppy mill?'" I'd heard the term before but didn't know what it was.

"In this country it's a big industry. I've heard estimates that there may be ten thousand here, and now we've apparently got one of these miserable places in our backyard." Grace was getting worked up about it. "Do you know that these people churn out more than five million puppies a year, sell them at eight weeks, keep them in wire cages exposed to savage cold and broiling sun, show them no kindness, and inbreed them so that they carry genetic defects? All you have to do is walk past their cages and they try to jump toward you to attract your attention. 'Bring me home' they seem to be pleading. The poor things."

"How awful. You've seen them before?"

"Yes, but not here."

"Are all the dogs sick, like these?"

"That isn't the half of it, Amy. The owners confine breeding dogs in cages for life, keep them pregnant, try to sell them when they wear out or put them to death."

What Grace had outlined about the miserable life of these poor animals was beyond belief. I had no idea that such abuse existed. I'd heard horror stories about chickens being confined, as well as cows and pigs and other food animals. I'd heard as well of cruelty to fur animals, but I hadn't known about dogs. The idea of such barbarism appalled me. I had a lot to learn. I vowed to go home and pet Molly when I left work.

"Where is this puppy mill?" I asked.

Grace shook her head. "I don't know. I think it's out toward Newtown, out in the woods. There may be hundreds of dogs confined out there. It's sure to be somewhere hidden because neighbors would complain about the barking."

"I'd like to see it."

"Don't try to find it, Amy; the owner may greet you with a shotgun. I can assure you that he doesn't give a damn about the dogs but may not want anyone to find it."

I vowed then and there to find it. I had to find it. I'd tell Ruth about it and ask her to go with me. We could pretend we wanted to purchase a puppy and heard he had some for sale. If the owner was in the business of selling dogs, wouldn't he welcome us onto his property with open arms?

I mentioned it to Dr. McDonald when he was carrying a dog from surgery. The dog was missing a leg and I'd been curious about it. Dr.

McDonald was now allowing me to keep an eye on the post-operative animals, where I monitored their progress and called a vet if there seemed to be any kind of a problem. It was a thrill to be entrusted with such responsibility. He carried this little dog as carefully as a baby. I'd come to realize that he was a kind and caring man who was tenderhearted to each of his animals.

"How did he lose a leg?" I asked him, looking at the bandaged stump; I was visualizing a trap or accident. A dog on three legs would have a difficult time maneuvering through life.

Dr. McDonald's jaw hardened. "This dog was in one of those puppy mills," he said. "I heard Grace describing them to you. She's absolutely correct about the dreadful nature of those places. This dog didn't even have a name, only a number; you can see it, 49, tattooed inside her ear."

I looked and, sure enough, there it was, burned inside the little animal's right ear.

Dr. McDonald went on, in answer to my question: "This dog has obviously spent her entire life in a metal cage—I've seen this before. So when the new owner put her on the ground for the first time in her life, her leg broke because it was so weak. There was no way to save it so I had to amputate it."

I stared at the poor little animal. "I'd like to shoot that man," I blurted out. "How could he be so inhumane?"

"The animal world is full of inhumanity, Amy. You never get used to it. I can't dwell on it because I couldn't function if I did. There are so many good owners, though. It's the bad ones that make you wonder about the human race."

During a brief afternoon lull, I asked Grace again about her experience with a puppy mill. Almost reluctantly, she told me that after her old dog died, she decided to buy another, so she and her husband Jim traveled to the next state where a breeder she'd heard about maintained a large kennel. The breeder was in a remote area, and she began to have qualms when she heard the dogs frantically barking as she and Jim came closer. Before entering, they had to wait for the breeder to return from a prayer meeting. Later she confessed that she found it ironic that this man prayed.

While they waited for the owner, they could hear the desperate barking of dozens of dogs kept in large sheds. When the owner arrived and showed them inside the first, they were horrified. They found dozens of wire cages, each holding a lonely and terrified puppy. These were the puppies for sale. Apparently the little animals were never let out, were filthy, and barely fed enough to stay alive. It brought Grace to tears.

Grace said she couldn't stomach going back into the second barn, so she sent Jim instead. In this second barn were the breeding dogs, which were kept eternally producing puppies. When Jim came out of the barn, his face looking ashen, he told Grace that some of the dogs were crowded into pens, trampling each other to reach him, just to touch him. Other animals in individual cages had gone crazy and were spinning around and around in their insanity. Some were injured, terribly ill, or near death. The animals lived in their own feces, unclean and mostly unattended. He said that the stench was unbearable.

Jim was shocked and sickened. When he suggested to the owner that the animals would be much healthier if they could go outside into fresh air and sunshine, the man retorted that the animals had no feelings and didn't mind being confined. Grace said that from that moment she decided to work in a veterinary practice to try to undo some of the evil that had been perpetrated on innocent creatures by cruel humans.

I realized then that I would have to somehow manage my feelings if I were to work around selfish and ignorant animal owners. If they behaved in such wanton ways toward animals in my care, how could I cope?

I talked to Dr. McDonald about it the next day, at a lull during lunchtime when he'd finished surgery. He was becoming a mentor, as was Grace.

"I'm not sure I can stand the way some owners treat their dogs and cats," I said. "How do you cope?"

He smiled and answered thoughtfully. "You can try to educate the owners, but most are wonderful people, Amy. They're not trying to make money from their pets; they have them because they love them. You'll see some of the most selfless people in here, utterly devoted to their animals. It touches your heart. It's the breeders for money, and those raising animals for the food chain, who break your heart. Animals are just commodities to them."

His words both cheered and depressed me. I'd have to try to be positive and not dwell on the inhumanity of some owners. But I remembered from Sunday school class that the Christian attitude was to care for all beasts, big and small. It was man's responsibility to help the weak. This was clearly a defining moment in my life, one in which I understood that I had a responsibility to stop cruelty to animals whenever I could.

I decided to tell Ruth about it. She wanted to be a nurse, and healing was her aim, too. Ruth and her parents lived merely a block away, and I loved to stroll to her neat Cape Cod house tucked into a shady stand of oak trees. "Come on over," she said when she heard my voice, so I did. Soon we were sitting on her porch, as we did so often, sipping iced tea in the cool of the evening.

"You wouldn't believe what I'm seeing at our clinic," I told her. "Two or three times a week owners are bringing in very sick dogs. It's almost like an epidemic."

"Where do they come from, Amy?" she asked. "What's happened to them?" She was as incredulous as I was.

"There's actually a puppy mill near here where the owner keeps his dogs confined in cages and never lets them out. The only time they're out of cages is when he tries to sell them at a mall. They don't even have names, they have numbers burned in their ears."

"My God, Amy. Where is this awful place?"

"No one seems to know. I asked the same question in the clinic. Grace thinks it's out near Newtown."

"But that's really in the sticks, ten or fifteen miles from a paved road."

"I know. I'd love to see the place where our dogs come from."

"So would I. Do you want me to help you? You've made me really curious. Such cruelty makes me mad."

I'd never thought about Ruth becoming involved. "Are you serious, Ruth? You'd come with me? That owner could be a maniac. Grace warned me about people like that."

"Hm. If he's selling dogs, he must have customers from time to time."

"I know. I've thought about it, too. Maybe we could pretend that we want to buy puppies."

"Of course. What owner would harass a potential customer?"

It sounded so sensible and logical that we fell for our own argument. We forgot that we might not be dealing with a reasonable man. Maybe we were crazy, but neither Ruth nor I could bear to think of the pain these dogs must suffer. We couldn't imagine any animal enduring such treatment.

But little did I know then that we would have a third to our little party: Rod Towns.

He called that evening after my talk with Ruth and asked me to have a beer with him at the Pub. "I'm tired of studying algebra, fractions and decimals," he said, "and need to clear my head. How about you? Will you come?"

"Sure," I said. I didn't even have to think about it, which surprised me, considering how I felt about him a couple weeks ago. But right now I needed to stop obsessing about the miserable animals at our clinic. Yet when he picked me up and we found a table at the Pub, I ended up telling him about the puppy mill, unable to get it off my mind. "It's somewhere near here," I told him. "We're getting sick and mutilated dogs at our clinic. They're weak from being kept in cages for so long."

"I can imagine. The owners must be nuts."

"I agree. I want to look at it with my own eyes. Ruth does, too."

"Where is it?" he asked.

"Near Newtown. No one seems to know where."

"But that's in rough country, Amy. I mean it. Moonshiners hung out there until the police cleared them out not so long ago. You and Ruth can't go out there alone. You don't know who's out there now."

I shook my head. "We're pretending we want to buy puppies. Nobody's going to bother us when we're potential buyers. We're not worried."

"Well, I am. You can't go there alone."

I was flattered but we weren't babies. "Yes, we can. We don't need protection. Besides, why would they bother us? There must be others buyers who visit out there."

"I don't like the sound of the place, Amy." He looked serious and concerned.

"We don't plan to hang out there, Rod, just make a quick visit. *If* we can find it."

"I'm going along, Amy."

"Rod, we don't need…" I was about to protest again, but the thought seeped into my overwrought brain that a solid-looking guy like Rod might be a welcome addition to our expedition, just in case.

"I won't interfere," he said. "I'll just tag along."

I took a swallow of beer and looked over at him "You really mean it, don't you?"

He nodded.

I almost laughed. "All right," I said. "Thanks for being worried about us."

"You're welcome."

A thought occurred to me. "Can you find out where the puppy mill is? Would the police know?" Wouldn't a budding attorney have a connection with police, especially if they knew where in the woods the still had been located? And especially if a large number of dogs were out there now?

"I'll find out," he said, nodding positively.

"Don't they need a license to operate a big breeding operation like that?"

"I'm sure they do, if they follow the rules. I somehow doubt that they do, but I'll look into it. When do you want to go, Amy?"

"Next weekend? I don't have any time until then."

He nodded. "The same with me."

"Good. I'll tell Ruth." For the first time I had a few butterflies in my stomach. Maybe we *were* acting in a rash manner. Probably we were. But I couldn't imagine any difficulty if we were simply looking at dogs for sale. Wouldn't they welcome customers? Dr. McDonald would know what to do if we located the place where all the sick dogs were coming from. It was worth a try.

CHAPTER EIGHT

A week to wait, but I don't have time to think about it. Today I'm filling in for anyone who needs me because Grace and Bets are off. In a regular office, I'd be called a "gofer." I like the variety of my temporary position because I get the chance to mingle with pet owners and meet their dogs. Usually they're very interesting and have a variety of experiences with their pets.

Today another dog purchased at the pet store in the mall has been brought to the clinic by its owners because of some kind of difficulty in its back legs. I sit in the waiting room with the couple, Mr. and Mrs. Kinkaid, and their dog, a Great Dane named Belle. The dog stands barely eye-to-eye with the diminutive woman sitting next to her who owns him. On the other side of the dog is the woman's husband, who is trying valiantly to hold onto the animal's leash. He is also a small person and appears in awe of his domineering wife. I am waiting to usher them into an examining room when Dr. Dubin is freed from his last patient.

Finally he signals me to lead the owners and their dog into the antiseptic room where he waits. He's a dedicated vet who sees his canine patients six days a week and loves every minute of it. He's the youngest veterinarian in the clinic, barely three years older than I am, and I'd love to ask him questions about vet school and veterinary practice, but I still don't know him that well. I like working with him because he's upbeat, likes to tell stories, and is a good diagnostician. He seems to me to have a gifted way with the animals in the clinic. He's also a nice looking man with chestnut colored hair and a smiling, confident demeanor. When they spot Dr. Dubin, Belle's owners seem to relax.

They declare that they have owned their dog only three weeks. Dr. Dubin takes one look at the condition of the dog, frowns, and says quietly to me as I'm collecting supplies, "It looks like we have another customer from the puppy mill." Except that it's easy to see that this dog is no puppy, but appears exhausted and has obviously been bred to death. In addition, the dog has some kind of problem with her back legs.

"Somethin's wrong with Belle's rear section," says the owner, Mr. Kinkaid. "She c'n hardly move it, ya see? It's slowin' her up big time."

"She can barely get up the stairs," echoes Mrs. Kinkaid. "We sort of lift up her hind section. We really can't do it much longer."

Mr. Kinkaid nods and looks at Dr. Dubin hopefully. "We're hoping you c'n do somethin' about it, Doc."

Dr. Dubin stands back to look at Belle. "Does she sometimes act almost drunk?"

Mr. Kinkaid thinks about it. "Drunk?" he asks, weighing the possibilities. "I wouldn't hardly say…"

"Drunk!" Mrs. Kinkaid interrupts. "That's just the way she is, Doctor."

Dr. Dubin looks from one to the other. "How about if you trot her around the waiting room," he suggests. "That way I can see how she moves."

Dr. Dubin, I know, is a patient man, careful and thorough, who has obviously taken an interest in this dog. I wait in the examining room for Dr. Dubin and the Kinkaids to return.

When they reappear, the Great Dane sits attentively between her owners. To me, they look like three peas in a pod—all similar height and attendant on Dr. Dubin's every word.

"Great Danes are prone to an ailment called wobbler's disease," Dr. Dubin announces. "It's a congenital, anatomical narrowing of the spinal canal in the neck and can cause decreased extension in both hips. It can come about when the dog doesn't have sufficient exercise or care. Luckily Belle doesn't seem to have hip pain. When you saw me turning her over to examine her feet, she didn't seem to have any trouble putting her weight on the top skin and not the pads. But when I put paper under her feet and slid her sideways, she splayed her feet as if she were on ice."

"There's somethin' wrong with 'at?" Mr. Kinkaid asks, voicing his concern.

"Both actions are abnormal," says Dr. Dubin. "Most of the time your dog doesn't know where her feet are, so she sways and appears drunk. Sometimes it can cause her to fall down."

Both Kinkaids look in alarm at the animal sitting contentedly between them. "Yep, that's the way it is," Mr. Kinkaid says, nodding sadly. "She falls right down."

"So what are you going to do?" Mrs. Kinkaid asks Dr. Dubin. She wants him to come up with an all-encompassing solution promptly.

"You should get the opinion of a veterinary neurology specialist and probably follow up with a spinal myelogram. I think you will then have a more definitive opinion. I can suggest…"

"A myelogram?" Mrs. Kinkaid asks incredulously. Her chin juts out. "I'll just ask my sister. She's a human neurologist."

Dr. Dubin shakes his head. "Human anatomy is entirely different from the anatomy of a dog," he answers. "One of our radiology specialists could easily determine if your dog is suffering from hip dysplasia or wobbler's. That will answer some of your questions about Belle's problems."

Mrs. Kinkaid takes firm hold of the dog's leash. "Then we'll just go along," she says, the interview ended. "We don't need any X-ray." She turns to her husband. "Come along, Harvey."

Mr. Kinkaid gets up from the chair where he'd been sitting. Both he and Belle trail along obediently behind Mrs. Kinkaid. Mrs. Kinkaid, I judge, is a woman who expects to be followed.

We watch them exit from the clinic. Dr. Dubin appears discouraged. "We'll probably never see either of them again," he says, a sad note in his voice. "And that's a nice dog. It needs help."

Vets are not as stoic as Dr. McDonald had indicated. Who could be? I'm thinking. "What will happen to Belle if she doesn't get help?" I ask Dr. Dubin.

"Belle's back legs will become significantly more painful and the disability will most likely progress to the front legs. It's a very debilitating condition. But the worst part is that it can be treated. I feel sorry for the needless pain that poor animal will suffer." He hesitates a moment, then says, "You need a sense of humor in this business, Amy. If you don't, you'll either leave the profession or go crazy."

Dr. Dubin is genuinely distressed, and I realize that there is a dark side to veterinary medicine, mostly brought on by humans. But since we are having a brief lull in the progression of patients, I asked him the same question I'd asked Grace. "What can an owner do if he or she buys an animal which is defective in any way?"

"Like that Great Dane?"

I nod. "We seem to be getting many unhealthy dogs here at the clinic. Grace says that they come from a puppy mill nearby. Is that so? And if I bought a sick dog, what recourse do I have?"

His answer is prompt. "You could activate the Pet Lemon Law."

"The Pet Lemon Law? You mean, like in cars?" It seemed unlikely that the same law which applies to faulty machinery could also be applied to animals.

"Exactly. Just like in cars."

What a novel idea! "How do you activate the law?" It wasn't exactly an idle question.

Dr. Dubin enumerates on his fingers. "First, the owner must save all documents regarding the sale of the animal, all vet records, then write down everything the dealer says. After that, he must call the Department of Agriculture and give them all pertinent information; they're the officials in charge. Next, he's got to inform local law enforcement and give them a sworn complaint. Anyone, like the puppy mill owner who violates any provision of The Pet Lemon Law, is guilty of a first-degree misdemeanor."

So the law does provide owners with rights! "Are puppy mills illegal?" I ask Dr. Dubin.

"Many are. Most have no permits. Even those with permits may be run badly if they aren't inspected regularly. Others are often managed by shadowy criminals. In my opinion, all of them should be put out of business." His answer is emphatic. He hits his fist against the palm of his other hand for emphasis.

I actually feel alarm. Is this the way it is in a veterinary practice? "Then why did you decide to be come a veterinarian?" I ask him, "with challenges like these? Don't they overwhelm you?" If I'm going to be a veterinarian, can I withstand these pressures? I'm not bulimic now, but I don't want to fall into that trap again.

"I love animals—all animals," he answers, rubbing his head in weariness—it's been a long day. "I'm even a vegetarian because I can't imagine eating animal flesh. We're all the same in this office. But the reason is really because of my brother."

I feel a story coming on. "Your brother?"

"He has cerebral palsy," Dr. Dubin answers. "He was depressed— said he couldn't find a good thing about his disability despite encouragement from everyone in our family. We suggested alternatives that required mental and not physical ability, but he wouldn't listen. He watched other kids walk smoothly across a room but his muscles wouldn't let him do it. He had operations on his feet, ankles, and even his eyes. Nothing worked; he'd fall constantly. His body refused to act normally, and his legs wobbled and buckled at all the wrong times."

I had immediate sympathy for the poor man: his physical problems were akin to my emotional ones with bulimia. "What did your brother do?"

"We knew that he was giving up, figuring no one would ever recognize that he was a person with any talent. But when he was 23, a miracle happened. A wonderful young Labrador named Sparky arrived at our door, a gift from Caring Canine Companions. He was a delightful, wiggly, enthusiastic little creature. His tail continually waved hello. We all loved him and my brother adored him."

"Did he work out for your brother?"

"The organization which presented him to my brother had transformed Sparky into a skilled service dog. He could pick up lost items from the floor, help my brother up and down stairs, bark on command, and open doors. He changed my brother's life. My brother went on to complete a master's degree at the University of Michigan, with Sparky assisting him to traverse the busy campus, helping him skirt icy patches, and even carry heavy books. Sparky still helps my brother, who now teaches physics in a university."

It was absolutely a miracle story.

Dr. Dubin paused. "There are many reasons I love animals. They're wonderful, diligent, helpful creatures. Sometimes I think people don't really appreciate them enough."

"I do," I said, thinking of Molly. "They save lots of people's lives."

That evening I sat with Ruth on her porch, drinking lemonade, and told her what Dr. Dubin had said. "It inspired me," I told her. "I'm really sure now that I want to be a veterinarian."

"Do you realize how much they help shut-ins and hospital patients?" Ruth asked. "Some nursing homes and even hospitals allow dogs to visit their patients regularly."

I'd discussed this with my Dad. He'd even seen dogs in a hospital wing where patients were ambulatory and recovering.

Ruth went on. "My Mom told me of one nursing home which kept a dog permanently to elevate the spirits of the residents." Ruth laughed. "On my way home from work today, I stopped by a pet store to pick up dog food for a patient being discharged tomorrow who won't have a chance to stop on the way home. Well, there was a man in the store asking if they sold rats for his pet python. Can you imagine? He was very upset when they told him they didn't carry python food."

"Ugh," I said, making a face. "A python will never make it as a companion in a nursing home. I hope I never have to treat a sick python."

"Would you have to?"

The thought almost made me gag. Then I remembered that Grace had told me about a vet who'd removed bullets from puppies, cleaned wolves' teeth, and reconstructed the mouth of a cat which had been badly burned by chewing on an electrical cord. "If others can learn those procedures," I said, "I suppose I can. But I don't know about a snake." I didn't know that my trial would come soon.

Ruth shook her head. "You're wonderful," she said. "I don't know if I could do it, Amy. You'll learn all kinds of new techniques."

"You, too, Ruth. Especially if you want to be an operating room nurse. I admire *you*." I helped myself from the lemonade pitcher Ruth had placed on the table between us. "Do you still want to try to locate that puppy mill?"

"Absolutely. I don't like to see animals mistreated, either, Amy. I want to find the place and see what they're doing. Who knows, maybe they're all right."

"From the looks of the dogs coming into our clinic, I doubt it."

"Does Rod still want to come with us?"

"I think so. I'll call him tonight. Meantime, he said he'd try to find out where it's located."

"Good. Let me know."

When I return home, I immediately call Rod. Luckily he's in, studying logarithms. He isn't in a very good mood. "Damn this stuff, Amy; this class is driving me nuts! Who cares what power a base is raised to, anyway? And why do I need to know the area of a parallelogram?"

I laugh at him despite his frustration. "Didn't you say there's a math section on your LSAT exam?"

"Unfortunately. Let's not talk about it. What are you up to?"

I relate the story Dr. Dubin had told me about his brother. "It really touched me, that a dog saved a life."

"Impressive," he says, "I still think you'll go broke becoming a veterinarian."

"You're insufferable, you know it? And offensive."

"I know. Say, I found out from a cop my father knows where the puppy mill is located."

"You mean it?"

"He's pretty sure."

"Good. You're still coming?"

"I wouldn't miss it for anything. I'd like to see where this scumbag holds out."

"He may be all right, Rod. Maybe my suspicions are wrong. But I doubt it."

"We'll find out, won't we? Want me to pick you and Ruth up Saturday morning."

"Thanks. Good luck with the logarithms."

He muttered under his breath something I couldn't understand before he hung up "Thanks. Good luck with the logarithms."

CHAPTER NINE

On Saturday morning, Mom expressed her concern about our foray into the woods. "I don't like it, Amy," she said. "I didn't tell your father because I know he'd have a fit."

"We're adults," I told Mom. "We'll be sensible. The owner of the dogs isn't going to chase us away. We're potential buyers."

"I don't trust people like that, Amy. Back in the woods, who knows where?"

"The police know where they are," I told her. "Rod told them where we're going."

"They care?"

"Yes, they do. They don't like people hiding out in the woods. Besides, we've got cell phones. Don't worry about us, Mom."

"If you aren't back in two hours, I'll call the police chief. He's a patient of your father's."

She didn't seem at all reassured, but just then Ruth arrived, having decided to walk to my house. She wore jeans and a sweatshirt because it was a cool morning, and had covered her hair with a scarf. I'd thrown on slacks and a heavy cardigan, and wore a loose cap. Minutes later, when Rod pulled up to the curb in front of my house, I saw that he wore a leather jacket. We were dressed for anything.

"Welcome to our big adventure," Rod said, opening his car doors for us. "You guys still want to do this?"

"More than ever," I answered. "But my Mom isn't too happy. I'm beginning to feel sorry I talked you both into this."

"But you'd go anyway, with or without us, wouldn't you?" Ruth asked. "Why should you have all the fun?"

I smiled at the notion of having fun. "I want to find out where those sick dogs are coming from."

"So do I," said Rod. "The cops would like to know more about them, too."

"I never even told my Mom what we were doing," Ruth confessed. "Anyway, she had the morning shift at the hospital so she wasn't around. And Dad, like always, is working at his office." Ruth's father was a busy CPA who frequently kept Saturday morning hours.

"Then let's get going," Rod said. We climbed into the car; I rode in the front seat while Ruth sat behind me. Rod unfolded a map the policeman had given him showing the approximate location of the puppy farm, and studied it for a moment. Then he started the car and nosed out into the road. "Incidentally, the cops do know where we're going. Richard, the policeman, put an X on the map—see it here. He even said to report back to him what we find out. The owner has apparently applied for a permit but it hasn't been granted yet, pending inspection."

Holding the map in one hand, Rod led us onto the main road, and then onto a small road, which went past the school and a motel. Five miles later we came a dairy farm, where several cows grazed contentedly behind a fence. After that, the road split and we found ourselves on a small road taking us past a nursery growing trees in front and plants inside a large greenhouse in the rear. Ten miles later we turned onto a gravel road leading into heavy woods. We were in the middle of unknown territory. Even if Richard, the cop, said he knew precisely where we were going, at this moment I wasn't reassured.

As the trees grew thicker, I felt my first real apprehension. It was obvious that not many people traveled along this road, although if the owner drove his dogs to the malls to sell them, he must use it often.

"I don't think there are people for miles," Ruth said. All we could see were trees and an occasional cleared area near a rundown shed or an abandoned house.

"If this map is right," Rod said, stopping to study it, "we should be almost there." He handed it to me.

I looked at it carefully. "I think so, too. But there isn't much detail on it."

Ruth was looking over my shoulder. "We're in the middle of nowhere." I detected a tremor in her voice.

But about a mile along the road, there was no mistaking the barking of dogs somewhere in the vicinity. A hundred yards later Rod pulled up before a fence enclosing a small nondescript house with a large truck beside it. Across from the house and down the road a short distance were several barns from which emitted desperate barking.

"My God," said Rod. "Do you hear that?"

"How can you miss it?" Ruth asked, leaning forward to see the surroundings more closely. "What's wrong with them? They sound… frantic."

I had a momentary impulse to ask Rod to turn around and drive away. But we were here because of me, and I couldn't give up so easily. I hesitantly got out of the car, planning to approach the house, when a man, dressed in dungarees and a soiled shirt, emerged from the house and stood gazing at us. He didn't approach very willingly and didn't appear friendly. "What'cha want?" he asked in a gruff voice, standing behind the gate, making no move to open it.

I called out to him. "We've come to see some of your dogs, sir. We're considering buying a couple."

"I sell 'em at the mall," he answered in a belligerent voice.

"Sorry, but we must have missed your sale," I answered. "Some friends bought several." And they're sick, I wanted to tell him. "We wanted to see others."

The man paused a minute, and his look of hostility softened. "You c'n take a look," he said, "long's you're already here. But I don't like people droppin' in on me unexpected."

"We didn't know how to get in touch with you," I said. "Our friends said you'd given them directions." In truth, it was the police who gave us directions, but I didn't want to tell him that.

The man thought about it, and the idea of making some money overrode his objection to our presence on his property.

"I got some young pups fer sale an mebbe some of my breeders. You c'n look 'em over if that's your aim." He unlocked the gate and we slowly walked inside.

He led us over the muddy, weedy yard to the nearest and smallest of the barns, a dilapidated structure, and removed a wooden bar to open the door. We slowly trailed Rod and the man into the first barn.

The interior was dark, lit by one lone bulb. What confronted us first, though, was the stench of dog feces and unclean animals emanating from the building. It almost made us gag. Ruth and I stared at each other, hesitant to go farther inside. But Rod continued through the door and we followed.

When our eyes became accustomed to the gloomy interior, we saw row upon row of wire cages, each one housing a single puppy trying desperately to reach us. It was the same scene that Grace had described. They flung themselves against the side of their cages, frantic to get out, except for one puppy, which lay on the bottom of its cage, spent and ill. Each appeared miserably forlorn, deprived of any human contact. It was pathetic and unnerving.

"These dogs seem desperate to get out," Ruth managed to say. "Don't they mind being caged so much, Mr..."

"Sidwell," said a woman, who had followed us into the barn. She glared at Ruth. "They don't mind being locked up. Animals ain't got no feelin's."

I'd heard that falsehood before. "Of course they do," I began. "All animals have feelings. These dogs are pathetic. Just look at them." I held my hand over my mouth and almost retched.

"You don't know nothin' about dogs," the woman answered. "We feed 'em and give 'em water. What else do they need? They're dumb creatures. Says so in the Bible. We heard it in church."

Rod could keep silent no longer; his voice was indignant. "What bible do you read, Ma'am? Dumb creatures doesn't mean stupid, you know."

Mrs. Sidwell shrugged, as if not caring.

Rod couldn't stop. "Do you mean to say that you keep these animals locked up in their cages like this all the time?"

"'Course," the woman said. "You let 'em out and they'll just run away. We got no time to chase 'em all over the county."

"Besides," said Sidwell with mock concern for his dogs, "We don't want 'em covered with ants or bugs."

"Of course not," said Rod in exasperation. "Especially when you want to get money out of them."

"Why else would I keep 'em?" countered Sidwell. "Don't tell me how to raise my animals!"

We were silent, at a loss how to answer these people.

"What's in the next barn?" I asked, almost afraid to ask. We had already realized that these dogs were mere commodities to the Sidwells, like potatoes or bricks. I could barely envision such a place.

"Breedin' dogs," said Sidwell. He ambled to the second barn, twenty yards from the first and larger than the one we'd just visited. He removed the bar across the front of the building, and we entered the gloomy interior, wondering what horrors we'd find inside. But I wasn't prepared for the cruelty of these people despite what I'd just seen.

Inside were more cages, some larger than others, with frantic dogs crowded into them, trampling each other trying to reach us. We slowly walked through the gloomy interior, examining each cage. There was shelf upon shelf of wire cages, where a few dogs had gone crazy and were spinning around and around like tops in their insanity, as Grace had described with horror in the puppy mill she had visited. Others were near death or maimed, lying in urine and feces on the floor of the lower cages: dogs in the tops cages defecated on those animals below. All were filthy, their coats matted and soaked, exuding a terrible stench. I had never seen anything so sad as those miserable creatures. It broke my heart. Ruth took my hand, and I knew that she was suffering as I was.

We walked unsteadily along the row of cages, nauseated and devastated. "Why are those dogs in the back so quiet?" Ruth asked, her voice unsteady. "They aren't barking like the others."

Sidwell's wife spoke up. "We don't want 'em barking. They make too much noise. We can't sleep at night.'"

"So what do you do?" Rod asked, peering into one of the cages.

"We fix 'em."

"You fix them. Like…how?"

"Easy," she said. "You jes' push a knife down their throats and cut out their barking box. Not hard at all." Hands on her hips, she gave us a toothless grin at the ingenuity she and her husband had used to solve their inconvenient problem so easily.

Ruth and I backed out the door, sick to our stomachs. I hadn't felt bulimic in months, but now I could feel a need to purge again. I couldn't stand one more word from these heartless people. But Rod wasn't about to be put off. "You have all this free land out here," he challenged, "and you leave these poor dogs confined in their wire cages for their entire lives? For years and years? They never see sunlight? Then you mutilate them. You call this humane?"

"Listen," Sidwell said, indignantly. "We got high marks from the agriculture department, the USDA. They said we was a 'model facility.' You wanna see the paper they give us, saying we're a good place? The best? Mister, you ain't got no right telling us we're not good enough to these dogs. I tol' you, they ain't complaining so why are you? We give 'em food an' water, and that's all they need."

Rod faced Sidwell and fought to keep his voice level and reasonable. "Mr. Sidwell, what if we were to give you money for a fence so these dogs could go outside? I'd even put it up for you. My friends would help."

"Of course," Ruth said, and I readily echoed her words. The idea of freeing these animals for even a few hours a week was immensely appealing.

"I tole you," Sidwell shouted, "I ain't spending no more money or time on them dogs."

"These dogs are no more than dollar signs to you?" I asked.

Sidwell stepped toward us. "You're gitten me mad," he said. "Now get off my property afore I throw you off."

I felt suddenly alarmed--I remembered Grace saying that we might be treated with shotgun pellets from some puppy mill owners. "Let's go," I said, taking Ruth's arm. Rod, too, had seen the possibility of this man turning violent. We turned our backs to Sidwell and walked hastily back to the car. Then we headed back down the road, our tires spitting gravel as we left.

CHAPTER TEN

We were so filled with helpless rage that we couldn't speak for several minutes. Finally Ruth said in a voice suffused with anger, "I sure hope I never see those people again. They're perfectly awful!"

I nodded. "Those poor dogs were miserable. I'd like to open the barns and let every one out."

"So would I," Ruth agreed. "But some of those dogs are too sick to go anywhere even if we did let them out."

"And if we freed them," Rod added, "we'd most likely be arrested and end up in jail."

Wait until I tell Dr. McDonald what we found, I thought. He'll be as appalled as we are. At least now we know where many of our sick dogs are coming from.

"Then what can we do?" I asked.

"I intend to tell the cops," Rod said. "They can't get away with this. It's legalized abuse. Maybe I can even get my father involved." For a guy who formerly didn't care much about dogs, Rod was becoming an advocate.

I'd been incredibly naïve to think that people like the Sidwells didn't exist. I'd imagined that they must have some feeling for their dogs. But they didn't. I thought of all the puppy mills which must exist around the country, housing thousands and thousands of sick and mistreated dogs. The thought devastated me. I told myself, you must do something about this, Amy; you can't allow those poor dogs to suffer. There must be laws which can stop such abuse and butchery. If there are, I'll find them.

This, I was well aware, was becoming a critical moment in my life. I simply couldn't go on without making an effort for those victimized animals.

We returned to my house. "Thanks for coming with me," I told my friends. "I couldn't have done it alone."

"It was pretty devastating," Rod acknowledged. "I'm glad we were together."

"And I'm glad we found those people," Ruth added. "They have to be stopped. I suffered for each one of those dogs."

We each nodded solemnly, a determined group. We had seen the pits of depraved human conduct toward helpless animals.

As Ruth, looking dejected, started to walk home, Rod called, "Hold on, I'll give you a lift," but Ruth shook her head. "I've got to clear my head," she said. "I've still got the smell of that place in my nose."

So did I; I knew how she felt.

"How about a beer tonight," Rod asked me. "I need a change of mood, too."

I readily agreed. We would meet at 7.

My mother had been waiting for me, worried about our visit to the puppy mill. Molly was at her side, sniffing at the unfamiliar dog stench on my clothes. "What on earth happened?" Mom asked, coming to the door. "You look as if you've seen a ghost."

I hugged Molly, rubbing the ruff at her neck. "I think I have," I said. "The ghosts of sad, sick dogs, imprisoned their entire lives in cages. It was the most sadistic treatment of animals I've experienced."

Mom shook her head. "How awful, darling. I'm glad you're home safely. I was worried about you. You can't tell about people like that, far out in the woods doing God-knows-what to innocent animals."

"I hope they won't be able to do it much longer. I'll ask Dr. McDonald for his advice and Rod will tell his father. I'll get in touch with the Humane Society."

Mom put her arm around me. "I'm proud of you, darling. But you know how hard it is to move governmental bodies."

I knew it but I was determined. "Did you know that Mr. Sidwell goes to church? The Bible says animals should be treated humanely. I remember it from Sunday School."

"And so does every other religion," Mom added. "But that doesn't mean that everyone reads the Bible. Or follows its teachings, either. There is more cruelty on this earth in the name of religion than you can imagine."

I told that to Rod that evening. We were having a sandwich in the Pub.

"I'm Jewish," he said, "and the Jewish faith goes right along with Christians. You don't abuse animals. I tried to tell that to Sidwell and that's when he threw us out."

"I'm glad he did," I answered. "I couldn't stand any more of that place." I had a thought, "Did you mention it to your father?"

Rod shook his head. "He's away on a business trip, so I'll tell him when he gets back. But my mother was shocked. 'Not many people know about puppy mills,' she said. 'Most people I know buy pure-blooded animals, which seem to be better cared for.'"

"And cost a lot more," I answered. "That's why so many people look for dogs at shelters. Often they're actually healthier. And pure-blooded dogs can be over-bred, too."

Rod nodded. "It's a nasty business."

"I can't wait to hear what Dr. McDonald says. He's one of the veterinarians at my clinic. Over-bred dogs are often sick and end up in his care."

Rod frowned. "At least this is keeping my mind off my math problems."

To his astonishment—and mine—I offered to tutor him, if he needed my help. After all, he'd pitched in to assist us to locate the puppy mill. "I'm pretty good at math," I told him. "I understand logarithms. If you need help, I mean."

He stared at me. "You're not kidding? You mean it?"

"Of course."

"I really could use some help, Amy."

"Then—how about if we meet at the town library? Monday afternoon after work?"

"Terrific. I'll be there. Thanks."

Monday morning I spoke to Dr. McDonald after surgery. First I told Grace that we'd found the puppy mill. "It's an awful place," I told her. "The dogs are sick and pathetic. It shouldn't stay in business."

She was astonished. "Dr. McDonald won't believe that you found it. He might have been upset if he'd known."

"Upset? Why?"

"Because he'd worry about your safety."

I looked at her. "It was my choice, Grace. I don't think I've ever done anything more important. That's what my friends think, too. We're going to report the Sidwells to the police and the Humane Society. Maybe the Society will remove the dogs to their shelter for adoption. Do you know, Mrs. Sidwell showed us a group of skinny, underweight dogs and said she was going to put them down because they were no good for breeding. Can you believe it, she was going to kill several of the dogs because they could no longer produce litters?"

"I can believe it, Amy. There is lots of cruelty in the animal world. You have to get used to it." Dr. McDonald had said the same thing.

"But," I vowed, "I'll try to do what I can to prevent it in my neighborhood."

Just then Dr. McDonald emerged from surgery, dressed in his blue scrub suit. Dr. Stokes, the second veterinarian in the practice, a tall man with the height of a basketball player, also garbed in blue, had obviously been assisting him.

"You won't believe this," Grace told the men, "but Amy located the puppy mill. She actually talked to the owners."

Both men stopped to look at me. Dr. McDonald removed his scrub hat with a swipe. "You mean it?" he asked incredulously. "How on earth did you do that?"

"The police told a friend of mine where it was located. We followed their directions and found it. It's the most miserable place you ever…"

I couldn't tell whether he was going to fire or congratulate me from the frown on his face. "Criminal types operate those places," he continued in a shocked tone. "You shouldn't have gone without the police, Amy."

"They were busy," I said. "My friend tried. They said they had other things to do. That made it our responsibility."

"What's going on?" Dr. Dubin asked, emerging from his office and hearing a meeting going on outside in the hall. He looked from one of the men to the other, then at me.

"Amy found the puppy mill," Dr. Stokes explained. Besides his obvious height, he's a redheaded, gregarious man who helped establish the clinic with Dr. McDonald. "The cops said they were too busy, so Amy took along a couple friends and found it in the woods near Newtown."

Dr. Dubin looked lingeringly at me. "That took a lot of courage, Amy. I'd like to get my hands on those people myself." At least he didn't sound upset with me.

"Do they have a permit for their unsavory business?" Dr. McDonald asked.

"The police are checking. They'll let us know."

Dr. McDonald stood contemplating me as if he were making up his mind what to do. "Come into my office," he said finally. "I'll talk to you while I shed my scrub suit."

Dr. McDonald suddenly didn't sound angry, but I still feared that I was on shaky ground. Yet Dr. Stokes smiled, which encouraged me.

Dr. McDonald led me into his office where he peeled off his scrub suit and washed his hands. Then he sat down behind his imposing desk and waved me to sit across from him.

"We all hate what happens to animals," he began. "But you can't take on the world."

"You can try," I said, still incensed by what I'd seen at the Sidwells' establishment. "I've never witnessed anything like that before. None of us could stand it."

"Who were the others with you?"

I didn't want to mention their names to get them into any trouble. "One is a nursing student and the other is going to law school. His father is a lawyer in Centerville."

Dr. McDonald nodded and started to get up when I remembered another of Sidwell's comments. "Sidwell said that his puppy farm had been commended by the USDA!"

At that, Dr. McDonald became incensed. "I doubt that," he said, emphasizing his words. "If so, the USDA isn't fulfilling its obligations. I'll personally write them a letter and tell them they're not doing their job. I'm getting pretty tired of all the sick animals coming our way.

Most of the work we're doing is *pro bono* because we can't bear to see these mistreated animals, but we can't keep it up much longer." He smiled. "Maybe we should send them a bill."

At least he hadn't fired me, but I figured I still wasn't out of the woods.

He slid a paper across the desk. "You may not be ready for this," he said, "but it's a national opinion poll from a cruelty to animals society. Read as much as you can. It's not easy reading."

It was a quiz. Question Number One asked if the reader was aware of the trade in dog and cat fur. It asked if we knew that animals killed for their fur were often dogs and cats, including puppies and kittens, stolen from their homes and often sold abroad.

The next question almost made me throw up. It asked if the reader knew that fur traders used methods including drowning, bludgeoning, and skinning alive to save money and avoid damage to the fur, and that dogs and cats can continue to breathe and blink for five minutes after they were skinned alive. The last question asked if "it is ever morally justifiable to kill animals so that their fur can be used and sold as clothing, furnishings, or trinkets."

I didn't have to think a second to answer that question, and Dr. McDonald didn't, either. "I'll notify the police, Amy. I admire your courage, but I'd stay away from places like puppy mills without police protection."

"Yes, sir."

He went on. "By hurting these defenseless creatures and allowing such legalized cruelty, we're hurting ourselves as a society—our souls, spirits, and sense of worth. When it's acceptable to abuse animals, it's easy to abuse each other, the poor, women, the environment, children, and any other vulnerable group. It can't be shrugged off as a necessary evil or be forgiven as a byproduct of big business." He paused a minute. "Sorry, I'm getting on my soapbox."

I admired my boss for his moral stand. "Then you won't fire me?"

"Whatever gave you that idea?" He laughed. "But I think I should give you more work to do to keep you out of trouble."

CHAPTER ELEVEN

The summer continued, and Dr. McDonald did write the USDA. The puppy mill was visited by the police, and mysteriously disappeared in the middle of the night along with the dogs and cages, leaving empty sheds. I knew that those pathetic dogs had been herded into a truck and transported elsewhere, to be imprisoned in another miserable locale. Yet Rod, Ruth and I felt vindicated for our action in visiting the place even if it caused Dr. McDonald's heart to skip a beat.

Veterinary Associates even gave me a party when my apprenticeship was over and I had to return to school. "You did a great job for us," Dr. Dubin said. "I hope you'll come back next summer."

"I'd love that." From thinking I was going to be fired to being asked to return was an incredible leap.

But my Dad was appalled and Rod's father was furious when they heard about our visit to the puppy mill. Rod related to me his confrontation with his father. "You think you can just take things into your own hands, mister?" he'd asked Rod. "Why, you'll get yourself and this law firm in trouble. I won't take you into my office if you behave in such an irresponsible way. You hear me?"

But Rod wasn't about to be put down. "Of course I hear you. We succeeded in getting the puppy mill closed. People are congratulating us."

"Well, I'm not one of them. Did that girl in the veterinary office put that idea in your head?"

"What if she did tell me about those crooks? You didn't see that place, Dad. It was awful. Sidwell was torturing those animals. It should have been closed a long time ago."

"What's it to you? You don't have a dog."

"Well, I'm going to get one."

"It won't stay in my house."

"Don't worry, I'll keep it at school. Incidentally, it was Amy who tutored me in math. She helped me get those terrific marks. I thought you'd be pleased."

"Well, I am. That has nothing to do with…"

"Yes, it does, Dad. She's a friend and I was happy to help her out. She certainly helped me. I'd do it again."

"I hope not."

Then, Rod hesitated. "Look, Dad, I don't care if you take me into your law firm or not. There are lots of other law firms. I have to live my life the way I need to live it. I can't live by your rules."

Incredibly, Rod told Amy, his father stopped and looked at him for a full minute before answering. "No, I suppose you can't," he'd said. "You're hotheaded, the way I was at your age. You'll get over it." Then he'd clapped Rod on the shoulder. "I rather think you'll be a goddamned tough attorney."

"It was amazing," Rod told Amy. "He sort of backed down. I never expected it. I don't know if I'll join his firm, and right now, I don't particularly care. I've still got a long time to go before I decide."

When Amy came to her father, she held a newspaper clipping in her hand. It mentioned that dog sales at the mall had been discontinued. "Don't worry, I've seen it," her father said. "And your mother already told me."

"You're upset?"

"Not about your foray, but did you have to get yourself involved with Henry Town's son. The father's a damned jerk and he's busy suing a colleague of mine."

"That has nothing to do with Rod."

"It's the same family, and I suppose the son will turn out just like the father."

"You don't know that."

"It's a tainted family tree. I've studied genetics, and the apple doesn't fall far from the tree."

I felt upset all over again. "That's really unfair. Rod's a friend and a good guy. He helped Ruth and me find the puppy mill. You're a doctor, Dad, and really care about people, so why don't you show more compassion for those abused animals?"

He thought about it for a minute. "I do care, Amy, but my colleague is going through hell. I care about him, too."

I wasn't going to argue with him because I knew his ideas were fixed, and because I loved him. His sympathy was directed toward his colleague and not the dogs, and since I knew I couldn't persuade him, I gave it up.

Going back to school involved the usual loading my car with collected books, clothes, and furnishings. Since the university was only 200 miles from Centerville, it was easy to get there in one day. Ruth was in my dorm, but she had a car full of belongings, too, so we drove separately. Hardest was saying goodbye to my parents and Molly. I told Molly to take good care of my grandparents, because they would watch over her for the time I was gone. My bulimia was gone, though with the despair I felt at the puppy mill, I was afraid it would return, but it didn't.

Rod and I continued to be good friends. His law courses kept him busy, as did my studies, but he had survived math. We met over a beer occasionally during the week, usually with Ruth. We were fellow conspirators, after all.

I continued with my veterinary classes, loving every minute. I also joined the Humane Society, volunteering on Saturday afternoons. And I became a pain to some of my friends.

One of the wealthy women students in the dorm showed up for a party wearing a fur coat—sealskin, she said. It was sleek, beautiful and warm. "My mother gave it to me," she said. "She moved to Florida and didn't need it any longer."

"It's so shiny and warm," I said. "I wonder how the seal feels without it."

She stared at me. "What on earth are you talking about?" she said. "What seal?"

I couldn't believe her detachment from the animal whose skin provided her comfort. "The one that was killed for your coat."

She shrugged. "I suppose it just died. There are lots of seals, you know. They just die."

"Really?" I said. "I doubt that your beautiful coat came from an old, dead seal."

"Little do you know," she answered. "Do you really think someone killed a live seal to get his skin?"

"That's exactly what I think. Hunters kill them with bullets, bats, or by skinning them alive. Did you know that they can blink and breathe for five minutes after they're skinned?" I was still furious about the cruelty I'd seen at the puppy farm and couldn't resist quoting the information from Dr. McDonald's national quiz.

"You're crazy, you know that?" she said, almost spitting out the words. "Stop telling me such awful things. I intend to wear my coat. You're just jealous that you don't have one."

I let it go. I certainly wasn't winning friends or convincing people. I felt sorry that she didn't believe me and that I was merely making her mad.

Most people didn't believe me. They did at a Humane Society I visited because they treated abused animals. Then I saw with horror in an old family album a picture of myself dressed in a rabbit fur coat on my way to church when I was a little girl. My mother bought it for me, and I thought it was the softest, most elegant garment I'd ever worn. Little did I realize how many rabbits had given up their lives so that I could own my magnificent coat. I didn't understand about animal cruelty back then, any more than the woman with the sealskin coat understood where her luscious wrap had come from.

"Does it bother you?" I asked Dr. Hanley one day after a class in cat anatomy at the university, "that so few people understand where fur comes from? They wear hats and mittens and coats without realizing that they're made by killing animals?"

"Of course it bothers me, Amy, but I think half our mission is to care for pets and the other part is to educate people. I even feel bad when I go into a restaurant and see lobsters trying to swim in water tanks with their claws tied with rubber bands, waiting to be boiled alive. I read something the other day which I copied down." He searched through some papers on his desk. "Here it is: 'An individual who knows the truth of animal suffering and of society's failure to address it, is harmed by both the suffering and society's disregard. He or she may then be taunted for being too tenderhearted.'"

"Then how do you stand it? What do you do to convey your grief for the animals?"

"I wish I knew, Amy. Mostly, as I said, by providing education and by being proactive. For instance, I didn't know how painful it was for a cat to have its claws removed, thus severing the delicate nerves and depriving the animal of mobility and defense, until I studied for veterinary school. It was like a human having his fingers amputated at the first knuckle. I was so ignorant. Then I published papers in veterinary magazines, assuming that others may not know, either. Also, citizen's advocacy led to California passing laws outlawing the mistreatment of ducks and geese by forbidding the practice of forcibly cramming metal feeding tubes down their throats three times a day to enlarge their livers up to ten times normal size so as to provide foie gras for restaurant patrons. Chicago also passed a law forbidding forced feeding of ducks and geese, even though the mayor called it the silliest law he'd ever heard of and vowed to overturn it. That remark led some restaurants to think they could continue the cruel practice. But the law held and other cities are advocating outlawing the procedure. You see, education can help."

Dr. Hanley went on. "If I learned one thing as a vet, it's that nonhuman animals are highly sensitive creatures who feel a wide range of emotions, just as we do, and some of their senses are more acute than ours."

I could only remember the Sidwells' comments that dogs don't have feelings. Every time I think of that remark, I get upset all over again.

CHAPTER TWELVE

I was back at school, and once again taking courses in biology, history, and math, as well as two in veterinary medicine. I was admitted to the vet school, hallelujah, having completed the necessary qualifying tests, gained the approval of the veterinary faculty, registered, and purchased the necessary books. Many who had watched with me through that one-way glass in the vet school last year were with me again. It was wonderful: I was even in Dr. Hanley's class. He looked tan, rested after his summer, and surprisingly eager to teach us neophytes the ropes of veterinary medicine.

On the first day, he explained what he called "blue-ribbon emotions" in animals, which he identified as exploration, rage, fear, panic, lust, care and play. These emotions, he said, are found in all animals, including humans. In fact, he said, when you dissect a pig's brain, you can barely tell the difference in the lower area from the lower section of a human's brain. This, he said, was the part of the brain where emotions originate.

He explained that when you electrically stimulate that part of the brain where emotion originates in any animal, human or not, it will react. If the part of the brain which governs anger is activated, that animal will bite. Humans stimulated in the same way won't bite but will also feel anger. If subjected to fear stimuli, flight will result. In the same way, activating the exploration system will cause the animal to start searching.

I really was astonished at the similarity between all mammals. I discovered that my dog Molly and I have lots in common. In addition, medications work the same way in non-human animals as they do in humans. For instance, Prozak will induce the same sense of calm in animals as it does in humans.

"Our reactions aren't all that much different from other animals," Dr. Hanley summed up. "Some people will deny it," he said, "because they're convinced animals are inferior to humans. Well, they're not. We're all God's creatures and we all have our place in the spectrum. Think what life would be like without the animals around us."

I could see the expressions on the faces of my fellow students as they imagined no longer seeing birds, squirrels, or their favorite pets. Without Molly, I wouldn't be here. On campus, I've seen Seeing Eye dogs leading disabled students to class. They couldn't survive, either, without their faithful companions.

Dr. Hanley had made his point with all of us.

Rod met me after class. We had continued our friendship, calling on each other for advice and companionship and enjoying an occasional beer. Sometimes Ruth, buried in her nursing studies, shook loose and joined us, but not today.

"How about a cup of coffee?" he asked. "I'm totally limp."

He did look limp. His eyes were tired and his dark hair hung over his forehead. "What's been going on?"

"We're having moot court arguments in law school. It takes a lot of research and preparation."

I looked at him curiously. "Moot court? What's moot court?"

As we walked slowly toward the coffee shop in the student union, Rod explained. "It's a simulated legal procedure, just as if you're in a trial. You have to debate a legal point just as if you were in court before a judge. I've been preparing for it since I returned to school."

Law was a strange new profession to me. "How do you prepare?"

"You study law texts from the law library to find precedents and facts relating to your case. Then you get together with your team and develop arguments either for or against the legal point you've been assigned."

"That sounds difficult, Rod."

"It's keeping me up nights."

No wonder he looks exhausted, I thought. "What point are you debating?"

He smiled. "Whether the Gun Free School Zone Act of 1997 violates the Second Amendment to the US Constitution. I'm arguing the affirmative position."

I looked at him and laughed. "I wouldn't know where to begin. Thank heavens I'm going into veterinary medicine." Then I laughed. "Although, of course, I won't make as much money as you lawyers do."

Rod hung his head. "I'm sorry I ever made that remark, Amy."

"Don't worry about it. I love what I'm doing. Don't you?"

He thought a moment. "I'm not so sure. My dad wants me to join his law firm so he'll have someone to take it over when he retires. It would be so easy to follow in his footsteps."

We ordered coffees, then brought them to a nearby table. I glanced at the solemn expression on Rod's face. "You don't have to study law, you know. There are lots of other interesting major subjects to choose from."

He made a tent with his fingers. "In that case, my father won't pay a nickel for my education."

"You're serious?"

"I wish I weren't."

I thought about it a moment. "What would you study if you gave up law?"

His answer was prompt "History. I love history. My history teacher is trying to persuade me to change majors."

"That wouldn't be too hard, would it?"

"I'd end up teaching. You don't make much money teaching."

"What's wrong with teaching history? My history teacher was a whiz. Is money all that important? I know you'd be a success at whatever you do, Rod. You're really bright and…"

"You don't know my father."

"You haven't spoken to him?"

"Not yet. I'll have to be sure first."

I nodded in sympathy. "I think you should do what will make you happy. I can't imagine spending my entire life doing something I don't like."

"I know, Amy. I envy you, being so sure what you want to do."

"Well, it was pure accident. I thought I was going to die, quite frankly. I'd about given up. I told you, my dog saved my life."

We walked back to class, and Rod smiled as if a weight had lifted. "Thanks," he said. "I feel much better. Back to the law books. For now, anyway."

"Get some sleep tonight," I said. "Forget the 'Gun Free Zoning Act' for one night."

He laughed. "I will, honest. See you tomorrow? Same place?"

"You bet."

Back in the classroom, a veterinarian named D'Allesio was teaching a class in autoimmune hemolytic anemia in canines. Dr. D'Allesio was a very tall Hispanic man who had a commanding presence at the front of the amphitheatre where we had many of our classes. He explained that this disease, called AIHA, causes a body to literally destroy its own blood cells. Antibodies, he said, stick to the red blood cells, which the body interprets as invaders. The immune system tries to attack the invaders but in the process injures the red blood cells as well. Dr. D'Allesio explained that hemolytic means destruction of the red blood cells and anemia is lack of red blood cells leading to weakness and heart problems. The condition usually leads to death of the animal.

Dr. D'Allesio then related an experience he had with a woman, Mrs. Wilbur, who arrived at the clinic in a flowered housecoat and worn slippers carrying a decrepit, nondescript black dog in blankets. The dog was clean, brushed, and very sick, with a rapid heartbeat and thready pulse.

"I told Mrs. Wilbur that he must stay in the hospital, and that his care would be very expensive, and that even after that care we might not be able to save Blackie." Mrs. Wilbur immediately removed a twenty-dollar bill from her pocketbook, saying she would pay the rest over time. As she left she called out 'God bless' and said that she would be praying for Blackie and for me.

"Well," said Dr. D'Allesio, "I thought that dog would be a goner, and that Mrs. Wilbur not only couldn't pay for our services, but was hoping for an impossible cure. When I tested and found that Blackie had AIHA, I called Mrs. Wilbur and, as gently as I could, asked her if she wanted to put Blackie to sleep because the disease was invariably fatal.

'No, Doctor,' the woman said, totally upbeat, 'you keep him overnight and tomorrow I'll get my prayer group going.'

"I was highly skeptical and thought that this dog was a no-win loser. But darned if the next day the dog didn't start to improve. His blood count was up and he sat upright in his cage. I phoned Mrs. Wilbur to tell her of the remarkable news.

'Oh, I had no doubt about it,' she said. 'You just keep it up and my girls will keep a'prayin'.'

"Within a week, that dog was busy eating and wagging his tail. I had no explanation for it, and still don't, but I understood then and there that healing wasn't just about textbooks and medicine, that it was a team effort involving the animals, me, God, and the people who love them. It was also about compassion, faith and serving others."

That, I thought afterwards, was probably the best lesson in veterinary medicine I ever had.

Then Dr. D'Allesio, with a smile, handed out a list he'd copied from an article by a wise woman named Joy Nordquist. Apparently he handed it out to all his classes. It listed all the things we could learn from a dog, including the following: (1) Never pass up the opportunity to go for a joy ride (2) Allow the experience of fresh air and the wind in your face to be pure ecstasy (3) When loved ones come home, always run to greet them (4) When it's in your best interest, always practice obedience (5) Let others know when they've invaded your territory (6) Take naps and stretch during the day (7) Run, romp and play daily (8) Eat with gusto and enthusiasm (9) Be loyal (10) Never pretend to be something you're not (11) If what you want lies buried, dig until you find it (12) If someone is having a bad day, be silent, sit close by and nuzzle them gently (13) Delight in the simple joy of a long walk (14) Thrive on attention and let people touch you (15) Avoid biting when a simple growl will do (16) On hot days, drink lots of water and lie under a shady tree (17) When you are happy, dance around and wag your entire body (18) No matter how often you are criticized, don't buy into the guilt thing and pout. Run right back and make friends.

I have that list in a special notebook and refer to it when I need a good laugh and a moment of truth.

CHAPTER THIRTEEN

Dr. Gregory, I became convinced, knew absolutely everything there was to know about cats. He was a short, jovial Irishman with a florid face and a quick wit. I looked forward to his every class. The amphitheatre was always full when he lectured.

During a morning coffee at the student union, where we often met to chitchat—almost as much of a ritual as it was with Rod--I told Ruth about Dr. Gregory. "He loves cats," I told her. "He loves their independence. He says they're easier to domesticate than dogs, though people sometimes think of them as wild creatures."

Ruth had just emerged from a class in the nursing school, an impressive four-story stone building behind us. It had been built forty years ago, Ruth said, and her mother had attended it, too.

Ruth nodded in agreement with Dr. Gregory's opinion of cats. "My cat, Barney, is really gentle. He's part of the family. He loves to sit in my lap, and purrs every time I pet him."

"He's a love," I agreed, having been chosen by Barney on occasion to provide a lap for his sitting pleasure. "Dr. Gregory says domestic cats haven't changed in appearance as much as dogs did when they evolved from the wild. He says you can't leash-train a cat easily."

"I never tried. But Barney never runs away."

I related to Ruth the morning's story Dr. Gregory told about cat loyalty in his own family. "When my parents moved to a new home five miles from the old one, their cat kept running away and returning to the old house," he said. "My parents had to go get him every time and bring him back to the new house. Finally it happened so often that the people living in the old house became attached to the cat. So when they offered to adopt it, my parents agreed.'"

Ruth laughed. "Cats are really loyal. When we found Barney, he was one of 40 cats living in a shelter. They lived in several cages where the doors were always open but they all slept together in the largest cage; that was their colony and they were attached to each other. Yet when I came to the shelter looking to adopt a cat, Barney came right over to me. That's why I chose him, because he seemed so independent, but it took us a few weeks to win him over to live with us. But when he did, he didn't want to leave us, either."

I asked Ruth about her morning classes. "Really interesting," she answered. "Actually, it was a course in basic body systems. Today we learned about the lymphatic system. That's the system that nourishes the body's tissues with red blood cells and plasma."

I contemplated the face of my friend. "You're so smart, Ruth. But I bet that your Mom is a big help to you. She's already taken those courses."

She smiled. "You're right. Mom explains what I don't understand. We're a great team." Ruth took a sip of coffee. "Say, what's going on with Rod? I saw him yesterday, and he barely said hello. It wasn't like him at all."

I nodded, having been privy to his concerns about law school. "He's not sure he wants to continue with his law studies."

"You mean it?"

I knew what she was thinking. "I suppose that his father would have a fit if he changed."

Ruth twirled a curl with her finger. "But don't you think he should do what he wants?"

"Of course. But it seems a hard decision for him."

"I can understand that," Ruth said, commiserating. "But what would he do if he didn't continue in law school?"

"He told me he loves history and would love to teach, but his father is putting him through law school and he feels obligated by that.

That's his conflict. And I gather that his father is a pretty persuasive character."

"He's probably the leading attorney in Centerville. I hear he wins most of his cases." Ruth thought a moment. "Listen, I'll talk to him when I see him on campus. He must have a free class around noon, 'cause that's when I run into him."

"He'd appreciate it, Ruth. I think he'll talk about it pretty freely with you because you're a good friend."

As it happened, returning from the coffee shop, I ran into Rod. He looked bummed. I almost passed him by.

I stopped and looked at him. "What's wrong, Rod? You look as if your world just caved in."

He motioned me toward a bench beside a fountain marking the center of campus. It was ordinarily a central peaceful place, with paths radiating out in all directions toward all the university buildings. "An hour ago I called my Dad on the phone and told him how I felt about the law. That I was having doubts."

"That couldn't have been easy. What did he say?"

"He said he was tired of my complaints. That I didn't know how lucky I was. And if I didn't shape up, I could forget about any help from him."

I couldn't believe Rod's father wouldn't at least talk the situation over with his son. "That's terrible! What are you going to do?"

"I don't intend to 'shape up' to his wishes. I just can't do it. So I just applied for student aid."

"You mean it?" I was astonished at the pressure Rod must be feeling and the decisions he was being forced to make.

"My father meant it, Amy, when he said he wouldn't support me in college if I quit my law studies. I know him and he doesn't make threats lightly."

"I'm so sorry, Rod. What did the aid office say?"

"They said they'd consider my request and let me know within a few days."

I nodded slowly. I had my fingers crossed for him. "That sounds optimistic. At least they didn't refuse you. You're already enrolled at the university here so they'll take you seriously."

"I hope you're right."

"What does your mother say?"

"She's pretty mad at my father. But she thinks I should stay in law school. Everyone in my Dad's family is a lawyer, so she's thinking about the family tradition."

"Huh! But maybe you really don't want to practice law. Your mother should honor that. After all, it's a lifetime decision."

"I know." Yet he looked slightly more upbeat, I thought, just having someone to unburden to. "It'll work itself out, Amy. Thanks for being in my corner."

I kissed him on the cheek. I meant it from the heart. But I had to beat it to class.

"I'll call you tonight," he said.

"Good. I'll be home studying all evening."

Dr. Gregory continued with his cat lecture, although my mind was on Rod's dilemma. I reflected on my relief and gratitude that my parents supported me in my decisions. My father had come to understand that I had no wish to become a medical doctor, and he wasn't haranguing me about it. I tried to concentrate on Dr. Gregory's words because his talk was both fascinating and my grades depended on understanding it. The class in the amphitheatre was hushed, also hanging on his presentation.

This afternoon he was holding an adorable little cat in his arms. "Cats can have what I call Lassie Moments, full of bravery and courage just as dogs do," he began. "This particular little cat, when he was a kitten, hated kids, the reason being that some kids frightened him so badly that he jumped out of a three-story window. Cats are extremely nimble so, believe it or not, he wasn't badly hurt and didn't need my services, but he was terrified. To make it worse, when the mother and her son returned home and found the little kitten, it had entered the cellar and was hiding behind a washer where kids, who had somehow entered the house, were throwing things at him. The cat never tolerated children after that.

'Another day the son was sick and staying home from school, when he heard a knock on the door. He opened the door and, being only 12 years old, didn't think to find out first who was there.

'Two neighborhood boys, who had been robbing younger children of their computer games, shoved the boy aside, entered the house, and began searching through his games. The younger boy demanded they leave but they laughed at him and continued plundering his possessions.

'Suddenly, the cat, which was pitch black and must have looked like a Halloween demon, came out from hiding, took one look at the intruders, arched his back, spit and screeched at the boys. They took off at top speed and never showed their faces around the neighborhood again. A witness said the boys streaked past him like Road Runner in the cartoon.'" Dr. Gregory felt that was a true Lassie Moment.

He told about another cat in his practice: "A woman who owned a Siamese cat reported that one night the cat came into her bedroom, jumped on the bed, and began meowing loudly. The woman pushed him off the bed but he wouldn't leave and continued his meowing. The woman finally got up, put him in the garage, but the cat continued his highly vocal cries. Finally the woman got up and let the cat out of the garage, but the cat immediately went to the sliding doors to the outside, meowing all the time.

'The woman realized that the rabbit hutch was in the backyard by the stream, but there had never been any trouble, even though rain had been coming down more than usual during the last week. She went to the hutch and saw that it was rapidly filling with water. She removed the panic-stricken rabbits one by one and saved their lives.'"

She told Dr. Gregory that her cat had never done such a thing before, but she understood that it had bonded with the rabbits after her daughter played with the rabbits and the cat in the yard. They became family and not prey. Dr. Gregory called this another Lassie Moment.

Then Dr. Gregory chuckled. "This is not a Lassie Moment, but I love telling this tale. It's about a cat which taught himself to use the toilet. The owner of the cat had noticed that on many occasions the toilet wasn't flushed, so she delicately asked her husband to flush after himself. Somewhat peeved, he declared he always flushed the toilet. So she spoke to their son. The son indignantly responded with the same answer. Things were tense around the house, she said, until one day she saw the cat using the toilet. She couldn't believe it. The only thing the cat hadn't taught himself was how to flush!"

Again I found the lecture funny, fascinating and instructive. Then I thought of Rod and reminded myself that not all of us were finding college life that easy.

CHAPTER FOURTEEN

Because I was worried, I called Rod. "How're you doing?" I asked him. "Are you feeling any better?"

"Thanks, I am."

"You were pretty bummed."

"I sure was. Ruth called me, too. I appreciate it."

"What are you doing?"

"Actually, I had an interesting class today—you know, the moot court thing."

I was astonished. "Then you decided to stay in law school?"

"No way. I'm going to apply for a change of major tomorrow."

"You mean--to history?"

"I already told my history professor. I called him at home."

I felt relieved, just knowing that Rod was embarking on a course of action which made him happy.

Rod continued. "My professor was really happy about it. He said he'd put in a good word so I could get on a work-study program and maybe even a scholarship. I'll have to work on Saturdays and some other times, but it's worth it."

"You've told your Dad?"

"Yes, and he's furious. I knew he would be. I had to hang up on him. But at least I won't have to take any more math courses."

It was a terrible situation for Rod, yet I managed to joke with him. "But you were doing so well. You're sure you don't want to continue with logarithms?"

He knew I was kidding him. "I hope I never see a math equation ever again."

"But you'll have to memorize dates."

"That's something different. I don't have any trouble with dates." Everyone to his own talents, I thought. I never could remember dates.

"Amy, my father may call you. He's pretty angry and he thinks you're to blame."

"W-h-a-t? You're serious?"

"I'm afraid so. I can't believe it. He thinks you're leading me astray. I know it's crazy, and I apologize. He wanted your phone number but I wouldn't give it to him. But he can get it if he wants to."

"You know I don't have any say in what you want to do."

"Of course I know that. I tried to tell him but he's really hardheaded. I'm terribly sorry. I told him in no uncertain terms to leave you alone."

The man was really starting to piss me off. "Don't worry about it, Rod. Maybe he won't even call. I'm glad you're feeling better."

But I wasn't. Who did this man think he was? But I wasn't going to let myself get flustered over it. Besides, I had studies to think of. I called Ruth to tell her of this latest wrinkle.

"You're not going to believe this," I told her, "but Rod's father is threatening to call me."

Her voice rose in astonishment. "He is? Call *you*? Why?"

"He thinks it's my fault that his son doesn't want to continue his law studies."

"You're serious? That's nuts, Amy."

"I think so, too."

"He's a little crazy, you know that? He wants to sue you or something?"

"Lord, I hope not. He must be a weird character."

"I think he's an angry man," Ruth said, "and trying to find someone to blame."

I thought about it a minute. "Well, I'm not going to let it make me sick, Ruth. I'm never going to go through bulimia again. It took me a long time to get over it and I don't want it back."

"You won't get sick again. I know it. Did I tell you that we studied bulimia in one of my nursing classes? You don't binge and purge, and your weight is normal. In your case I think it was brought on by your brother's death. That was a terrible shock and might have made anyone sick."

Her good words raised my spirits. "Thanks, Ruth. And thanks for talking to Rod. He said we cheered him up."

"Good. He just needed someone to talk to."

After class I bought a hamburger at the student union, brought it home, made some tea, and began studying for a math test. Then the phone rang. It was probably Rod or a friend on the other end of the line, but Rod had warned me and I answered the call with misgivings.

I was right to have misgivings: it was no friend; it was Henry Towns, sounding barely under control. "Miss Richards," he began, 'I'm sure that you are a very nice girl or my son wouldn't consider you a friend, but what the hell are you doing trying to talk him out of law school?"

My stomach felt hollow as I tried to summon my responses. "Mr. Towns," I began, " I never tried to talk Rod out of law school. He told me he wasn't enjoying it, so I listened to him. That's all I did. He said he loves history. He'd like to teach…"

"Don't try to tell me what he loves. I'm his father. He loves the law and your interference is completely unwarranted. He plans to join my law firm, the firm of my father and grandfather. I've given him every advantage, helped him to plan his future course…"

"But Rod says he doesn't want to be a lawyer. Have you spoken to him?"

"Of course I've spoken to him. I find your meddling completely inexcusable. I demand that you stop talking to my son."

"Stop talking…? With all respect, sir, isn't that Rod's choice? Rod's a friend. I tutored him in math last summer so he could continue his law studies."

"A lot of good that did, didn't it? Now he wants to quit."

"Mr. Towns, Rod's very bright. Don't you think he should be allowed to take whatever courses he chooses?"

"A history teacher! Huh, I hear you want to be a veterinarian. Your father's a doctor. See, I know something about you…."

"What does that have to do with Rod?"

"If you had any brains you'd choose a profession that'd make you some money."

"Is that was this is about—money? And joining your law firm to make a pile of it?"

I could hear him take an angry breath. "Miss Richards, I'll guarantee that if you pursue my son, I'll get a restraining order against you. You'll be sorry you took this path!"

"But I never pursued Rod. I told you we're just friends…"

But he'd slammed down the phone.

I was quivering. I hung up the phone, feeling as if it was made of lead. I didn't know what to do. I called Rod.

He wasn't in, but I left a message on his answering machine. "Your father just threatened me with a restraining order, Rod. He thinks I talked you into changing majors. He's furious that you aren't following the family tradition and thinks I'm to blame. Please call me."

Then I called Ruth. "Ruth, I just got a phone call from Rod's father."

"No! What did he say?"

"He threatened me with a restraining order if I talk to his son ever again. Can you believe it?"

"No. I can't, Amy. A restraining order!"

"What right does he have to threaten me? I haven't influenced Rod. But if talking over his plans is a legal case, then I'm guilty."

"You're not guilty of anything." I could hear her voice rise in indignation. "He's got a lot of nerve. Mr. Towns wants to select his son's friends? What an overbearing prick!"

"Do you think I need to get an attorney, Ruth? It'll be expensive for me… "

"And Towns knows it. But I think he wants to intimidate you. He must know half the legal establishment in town."

"That's what I'm afraid of. He knows he has the advantage."

"But that doesn't mean he can get away with harassing you. Towns is just a hothead. Have you spoken to Rod?"

"Not yet. I'm sure he'll call back soon."

I started to calm down; talking to Ruth was very reassuring. "I can understand why Rod found it so hard to change his major, Amy. Can't you?"

"I sure can."

"Let me know when you hear from Rod, okay?"

"I will. And thanks."

But I still had a math test to study for. If old man Towns didn't have anything better to do than harass me, I sure did. That test was a final in the course and I wasn't going to blow it because of Rod's father.

Still, I decided to call my mother, who must be home by now. She usually left work at the library at 5:00 and it was now 6:00.

"Hi, Mom," I said, feeling guilty as if I were about to drop a bomb on her.

"What's up, Amy?" She always astonishes me because somehow she can tell by my voice when something is wrong.

"Do you remember my friend, Rod Towns?"

"Of course. You tutored him all last summer." She hesitated. "He's flunked out?"

"No, Mom. His father threatened me with a restraining order if I ever see him again."

There was a long silence. "Amy, what have you two been doing?"

I almost laughed and somehow it broke the tension. I know she remembered that we found the puppy mill, and that she was conjuring up all kinds of transgressions. "Mr. Towns thinks I talked his son out of law school."

"*What?*"

"It's not true, Mom. Rod decided to change his major from law to history and all we did was talk it over. It's true, I encouraged him when I knew how he felt. I'm a friend, after all. Mr. Towns thinks I'm responsible. He wants Rod to follow him into the family law business and Rod doesn't want to do it."

"How could Towns possibly think you're responsible?"

"I don't know. It was Rod's own decision. Rod's history teacher thinks it's a wise decision because he's so talented, and has been pushing Rod to transfer his major."

"Towns is going to threaten Rod's teacher, too? For interfering with his son's decision?"

It was ludicrous. "He wouldn't go that far, Mom."

"Keep your chin up, Amy. I'll talk to your father about it, but I'm sure he'll think it's ridiculous, too. Henry Towns has the reputation of being a bully."

"I agree. I'll let you know what Rod says."

"Please do, darling."

CHAPTER FIFTEEN

Rod called that evening. "What the hell did my father say to you, Amy? He threatened you with a restraining order? Why?"

"He doesn't want me to see you ever again, Rod. He thinks it's my fault that you want to change your major."

"What? I'll straighten him out, Amy. He's not going to interfere with my life, or with yours, either. I've really had it."

"I've been thinking about it, Rod. There's not much he can do to influence you when you've made your mind up."

"You're right about that."

"Can he really place a restraining order on me?"

"He can do anything he wants, but his colleagues would laugh him out of court. And I'd testify that his accusation is wrong, and get a restraining order against him." He paused. "Listen, are you all right?"

"I'm feeling better—but he did scare me a little. He has a way of intimidating people."

"Tell me about it! But it's mostly bluster. Say, do you feel like a beer tonight?"'

"After finals, Rod. I've got math tomorrow, and my last vet quiz the day after. I can't believe our semester is coming to an end."

"Neither can I. But it's been kind of wonderful, deciding on history. As Santayana said, Those who don't know history are doomed to repeat it. It's always meant something to me…and now maybe I can concentrate on what I love best."

"It's obvious to me that you do love history."

"I intend to talk to my father tonight. Please don't worry, Amy."

I hit the books again, still worrying despite his advice, but I was sliding through trigonometry review when my father called. "Amy, your Mom already told me. If that weasel Towns calls you again, I'll go see him and break every bone in his body."

My dad could do it, too, because he was a boxer in college and captured the intercollegiate boxing title his senior year. "I think it'll be all right, Dad. Rod has already changed his major to history and he won't change it back."

"You realize that Towns is suing one of my partners?"

"Mom told me. Rod says that his father sues lots of people just to scare them."

"What a dirty trick! Those people then must spend money to defend themselves."

I agreed with my father; what's more, I sympathized with each of Towns's victims.

"Your mother and I are here for you, baby. Don't worry about that. Just let me know if you hear anything more from Towns. I'll go talk to him."

"I don't think talking will help, Daddy."

"You may be right, but I'm not going to let him intimidate you anymore, and that's final."

It was great to have my father on my side. Usually he's mild-mannered but he can be very forceful. I could tell by his voice that, with my brother gone, he wasn't about to let anything happen to me.

I decided to go study at the library, to get away from the distraction of the telephone. Every time I heard one ring nearby in our dorm, I jumped and lost my train of thought. At least the library was quiet.

While reviewing a chapter in my beginning veterinary book, I happened to see an introductory chapter on cows, immediately following the chapter on cats. Curious, I read a few pages. One veterinarian wrote that he had to flunk five applicants during audits by the American Meat

Institute in 1997 because they didn't live up to a humane treatment of animals. These automatic fails were the result of applicants hitting or beating an animal up, dragging a live animal, driving animals on top of each other on purpose, sticking prods and other objects into sensitive parts, slamming gates into them, or yelling at them. Apparently cattle, like many animals including humans, are afraid of angry people. I can understand that, having been recently intimidated by Henry Towns.

Who, I wondered, would do these things to animals on purpose? Plenty of animal handlers, I guessed, if there had to be rules against such cruel practices. I decided at that moment that I would be a small animal vet, because I couldn't stand mistreatment on such a large scale. Small animals are mistreated, too, but at least you could stroke them.

When I returned from the library, there was a message on my answering machine from Rod. So I called back.

I was on tenterhooks. "I just spoke with my father, Amy."

"And...?" I was actually trembling.

"He says he won't pay for my education. He said that's final. He turned me loose; he said I'm on my own."

I could hardly believe it, but it was what Rod had been expecting.

"But I think I'm going to get the scholarship. My history professor spoke to the committee and they seemed receptive. At least I'll get my father off my back."

What a shame, I'm thinking; it was a no-win situation for both Henry Towns and his son. Towns will lose a son because of his pigheadedness and Rod would lose contact with his father. In addition, he'd be deprived of financial support.

"I'm so sorry, Rod. Was he angry?"

"He was raging. So was I."

What a scene that must have been!

"But he didn't say a thing about you, Amy. I think you're off the hook."

Maybe. Henry Towns could change his mind in a minute. But it was obvious that Rod would have to work his way through college, which would take both time and added expense.

"The only consolation is that you've made your decision, Rod. That was painful."

"Thanks for your help, Amy. We're still going to have a beer tomorrow night after your exam?"

"I can't wait."

I was still shook up by Henry Towns's threats, but my math exam was scheduled for 9 a.m. tomorrow morning and I had to concentrate on that. In spite of all the interruptions, I knew math cold. I wasn't worried about veterinary medicine, either. I had already been taking introductory courses; next semester I'd start studying the basics of animal anatomy, and would have to start cramming more intensely. I couldn't wait.

Ruth was cramming, too. When I called, she was in her study cocoon, as she called it: her shades were pulled, she said, and she had a "no admittance" sign on the door. "I'm getting there, Amy. Can you make it for a beer tomorrow night? Rod said he'd called. Any more studying will drive me crazy."

"I can taste the beer already. Are we going home together for spring break after last class."

"I'd love it. My mom said she'd meet us."

I wanted to see my parents—and Molly. My grandparents were still away. I had to tell Molly that I knew much more about her than before I went to the university, that I could listen to her heartbeat, palpate her inner organs, take her blood pressure, and talk to her intelligently about canine diseases even if she didn't understand a word. I knew she'd wag her tail appreciatively.

We managed to survive exams and met at The Pub for the promised beer. "What are you going to do during break?" Ruth asked Rod as we three shared a pizza and drank beer. "Go home? See your parents?"

"My dad will be in Las Vegas for a convention. Just my Mom and brothers will be home."

"What luck!" I said. "How does your Mom feel about all this?"

Rod traced the cold condensation on his glass with his finger. "Unfortunately, she's under Dad's thumb. But she sent me money to clear my bills for the semester, and I'm sure Dad doesn't know it."

"At least your Mom understands," Ruth said.

Rod nodded, then looked at me. "You're going to work at the clinic during break?"

I nodded. "They even offered me a job again for summer."

"And I'll be at the hospital," Ruth added. "They're really short-handed."

"Congratulations," Rod said. "Jobs aren't easy to get."

"What will you do?" Ruth asked.

Rod knew that his father wouldn't allow him at home, nor would he want to live there.

"Construction at the park, I hope. The town wants to build a gazebo and a storage building. I've already applied."

"You can find a place to live?" I asked.

"I'm looking around," he answered. "There seems to be lots of housing for rent. Other people are looking, too, so maybe I can team up with some other guys." He actually sounded upbeat despite the confrontation with his father. Maybe good things can come from adversity; I got well, thanks to Molly, when others feared I might die. I'm studying in the vet school and am happy now with what I'm doing.

"Then we might all be in Centerville this summer," Ruth said.

We all nodded: happily, the three musketeers would carry on.

Spring break went too fast. It was wonderful to see my parents, to rub the ruff around Molly's neck, and to have her sleep next to me at night. Dr. McDonald, Dr. Dubin, and Dr. Stokes greeted me with enthusiasm, said they were terribly busy, and put me to work right away registering patients and taking charge of the kennels.

I loved caring for the boarding dogs and those recovering from surgery. One case was hilarious—at least I thought so. Mr. Selnik, a 70-year-old, had a Doberman, Fritz, which Dr. McDonald thought should be castrated if Mr. Selnik didn't want his animal urinating on the furniture, wandering away from home, or impregnating female dogs.

"You can't do that to my dog," yelled Mr. Selnik. "Cut off his balls? Then he won't have his manhood." He thought about it a minute, then said," He won't squat to pee like a sissy dog if you de-ball Fritz? He'll raise his leg?"

"You're right," said Dr. McDonald, barely suppressing a smile.

"Then do it, dammit," said Mr. Selnik.

But after the surgery, Mrs. Selnik called Dr. McDonald to report that Fritz was depressed and so was Mr. Selnik. When they arrived at the office for a conference, Mrs. Selnik said, "You can understand how Fritz feels—he knows something's missing. But my husband"—she pointed to Mr. Selnik—"still has his and they work fine. You've got to do something about Fritz, because my husband is so embarrassed he won't even take him for a walk, and they both used to loved it."

Dr. McDonald suggested that he could surgically insert silicon prosthetic testicles called neuticals into Fritz's scrotum, which would not function but would look authentic. Mr. Selnik thought the suggestion to be a fine idea, while Mrs. Selnik threw up her hands and said she'd never heard such an outrageous idea, but she'd agree to it if that's what it would take to make her husband happy. Before I left the clinic to return to school, Mrs. Selnik reported that the surgery had worked fine and that Fritz and Mr. Selnik had resumed their walks, strutting their stuff, and that peace had at last been restored in their home.

"We look forward to having you here this summer," said Jeff Dubin, smiling and stopping to talk to me. "How are things going at the university?"

"Really well. I love studying animals. It's the right field for me."

"Good for you. It'll be nice to have you around."

"Thanks."

"Maybe we can get better acquainted. I'll try to help out whenever I can."

I was energized by his remark. I liked the clinic and Dr. Dubin, and already looked forward to this summer.

And, I thought, it would be wonderful to be home.

CHAPTER SIXTEEN

My spring veterinary studies were tough, but I didn't expect that they'd be easy. I had continuing classes in chemistry, cell biology and animal anatomy, and knew that next year I would delve into medications, neuroanatomy, and parasitology, among others. Next year, I estimated, would be even harder.

Rod did get his scholarship, but he still had to work on weekends in one of the big university kitchens, but he didn't seem to mind it. He was immersed in modern history and in classroom teaching techniques. "History is not so far off from law," he declared, "because law is based on legal precedents which are rooted in the past. That's what I like about history: it's the basis for everything in human existence. It *is* human existence." I was impressed with his enthusiasm. He wasn't looking back.

Ruth had decided that she wanted to learn how to assist in operating rooms, which would take longer than she'd originally planned, but the study fascinated her. It began to seem as if we were all going to spend the rest of our lives in school.

"Have you considered," I asked Rod and Ruth one weekend when there were no classes and we could share a pizza in a local campus hangout, "how long it will take us to finish our education?"

"At least they lowered tuition costs," said Rod. "That helps a lot. If I'm going to spend my life in school, at least I have enough left over so I can eat."

Ruth laughed. "You'll be able to student tutor before long, won't you? Won't they pay you a little?"

"Not much, but every little bit will help," he answered with a smile. "Maybe then I can give up some work hours in the kitchen. I won't miss it."

"Wish I could tutor some students, but I don't have time," Ruth answered. "It would help my poor suffering parents pay for my education."

"Amen," I echoed. "But, bless their hearts, mine aren't complaining."

"Did I tell you?" Rod said, making a wry face, "that Mom called and said my father wants to come visit? He intends to just drop in when he has free time."

I was aghast. "Why?"

"Mom said he intends to knock some sense into my head before it's too late."

Henry Towns wasn't giving up! "When do you think he'll come?" I asked.

Rod shrugged. "Who knows? If I did, I'd spend extra hours at work."

"Why doesn't he just stay home?" Ruth said. "Hasn't he caused enough trouble already?"

I agreed. It didn't seem as if Towns had reconciliation with his son as motive for his sudden visit; rather, he was going to browbeat him into returning to law studies. He was obviously determined to coerce his son into the Towns law offices at any cost.

Actually, two weeks later, just before final exams, Henry Towns did come to campus to belabor Rod. Luckily, Rod had drawn fewer hours in the kitchen so he didn't have to contend with studying and his father at the same time. They met in a swank restaurant near campus, and Rod said everyone in the restaurant could hear his father's closing arguments about returning to law classes at the top of his lungs. "It was embarrassing," Ron told Ruth and me when we met after class. "Some of the patrons turned around to look at us, and the maitre d' came by our table and requested that he keep his voice down."

"It must have been awful," Ruth agreed.

"But the worst of it was that he went to the dean of the law school and asked him to pressure me into staying in law studies."

I held my breath. "What did the dean do?"

"He refused to go along with my father. He called me in, we had a nice chat, and I told him I liked history and intended to stay in my major. He said, that was fine and good luck. He's a very nice guy."

I heaved a sigh of relief for Rod. Ruth said, "I'm glad it turned out all right, Rod. Then your father went home?"

He nodded. "He wasn't very happy, but I don't think he'll pester me again."

I hoped he was right.

The end of school came six weeks later, and I returned to the clinic, Rod began his construction job at the park, having found a place to rent for the summer, and Ruth worked again at the hospital.

Back again at the clinic, it seemed as if I had been advanced in my duties, beyond taking care of dogs in the pens. Jeff Dubin even let me observe his simpler surgeries. Several times he even asked me to suit up and help by holding the animals. Fascinated, I watched him remove a ball from a dog's stomach. Jeff explained that the dog, a cute Lhasa Apso, had been vomiting severely during the past week, and an x-ray of its abdomen clearly showed a ball, which the owner thought the dog had swallowed as long as three years ago. I was astonished when Jeff showed me the x-ray picture, which clearly revealed the shape of the ball. He determined that it should be removed immediately.

I was suited in surgical scrubs and a mask just like Jeff's. After he anaesthetized and prepared the little dog for surgery, he explained what he was doing. First, he took his scalpel and made an incision into the dog's abdomen, stopping bleeding as he went. Then he groped with his fingers inside the incision, located the stomach, and isolated the ball. It was clearly visible through the stomach tissue. Then, he made a second incision through the stomach wall into the stomach itself, and grasped the ball with forceps.

Astoundingly, it was one and one-half inches wide, and looked terribly deteriorated. How the little dog had managed to swallow an object that large was a mystery to both of us. And that the ball stayed in the dog's stomach for three years without killing the animal was beyond my comprehension. But Jeff explained that he'd successfully removed all kinds of articles from a dog's stomach before, including a sock and hairbrush, without incident. Luckily, Jeff said, this dog's stomach wasn't infected from having carried the ball around for such a long time.

Later, he sutured the wound with what he called an inverting continuous suture and said that a dog's stomach is filled with blood vessels and therefore would heal rapidly. The dog's owner actually kissed Jeff in the waiting room when he said her dog was doing well and would be running around soon.

I was absolutely overwhelmed with what I'd seen. Jeff, in my opinion, was a highly trained magician. I hadn't a clue how I'd learn all those techniques, but maybe one day I would. I was determined to try.

One Saturday, Jeff had a call from a nearby snake breeder, telling Jeff that his corn snake was eggbound, and hadn't been able to deliver at least two eggs. "I think she's gonna die, Doc," the breeder said, "if that egg isn't removed. I've massaged her and nothin's working. I'm afraid it's up to you if I'm gonna save Twistie."

"That's the snake," Jeff explained in answer to my puzzled look. "Can you help me out? Both Grace and Bets are gone, Avery has the weekend off, and Warren's at a wedding."

"S..sure," I stammered, "I guess." Up to now I'd made every effort to avoid snakes, finding them, to tell the truth, horrifying.

A half-hour later the snake breeder arrived with Twistie in a little round basket and placed her in Jeff's custody. Jeff didn't seem hesitant about this at all, acting as if he were an old hand at handling reptiles. No doubt he was. I suppose I've got to learn sometime, I told myself. Up to now, I'd pictured myself handling cats, kittens, dog and puppies, not wiggling, slimy snakes. Yet Jeff calmly examined Twistie, actually picking her up and maneuvering her around in his hands.

"We'll have to get the operating room ready," Jeff said, telling Jim, the remaining orderly, to bring out a wooden slab to use as the snake's operating table. "A metal table will drain heat from her body," Jeff explained. Then he prepared to anaesthetize Twistie by placing her in a box and administering gas through a valve directly into it. I'd never seen anything like this before, and when the snake was sedated, I was shocked when Jeff said, "Now will you wash the snake's skin, please?"

Before I could react, he handed me a pad saturated with antiseptic and indicated where I should clean Twistie's body.

Taking a deep breath, I touched the pad to the snake's skin, then discovered that I must hold the snake's body with my other hand if I were to apply pressure. At least the snake wasn't awake!

To my astonishment, on touching the snake I discovered that the skin wasn't cold or slimy but felt warm to the touch. Reassured, I cleaned with more vigor.

"Now I need to position drapes," Jeff said, tucking a sterile cloth over Twistie, and fastening it with material that looked like masking tape. Jeff examined the drapes critically, then said, "Now I think we're ready to begin."

He reached for a scalpel and made an incision on the snake's body. "You see this raised area," Jeff said, pointing to swollen-looking section of Twistie's midsection. "That's where the eggs are hung up. They've been there for three weeks, so we might have a little difficulty."

He continued to carefully cut through the snake's skin. "We must avoid cutting the ventral vein in snakes," Jeff continued, talking to me as if taking me into his confidence. "Now, through this incision, you can just see the first egg." With forceps, he maneuvered the egg carefully until he managed to pull it through the incision. To me, it looked like a slippery, soft brown ball.

"That's the egg?" I asked. "But it looks so large."

"It *is* large," Jeff said. "And this poor reptile has two more like it inside its body. I'm going to try to express all three through this one incision so that I don't have to make another."

Jeff bent over the snake and was finally able to prod the other two eggs, one of which was broken, from Twistie's body. Jeff positioned the three eggs, side-by-side on the drape, then examined each of them with his surgical glove. "She'll feel a lot better now," he said. It fascinated me that he was talking about a snake and not a dog or cat; I'd never thought before about how a snake felt. From now on, I would.

Jeff closed the snake's body and Jim took Twistie into the recovery room. Jeff looked at his watch. "Nine o'clock. It's been a very long day. I'm famished. Would you like to get a bite with me? There's a small Italian restaurant behind the clinic."

I wasn't even aware that I was hungry until Jeff mentioned it. Then I was suddenly starving: I hadn't eaten since noon. "I'd love it," I acknowledged. But I also realized that the thrill of eating with one of my bosses, and a handsome, talented one besides, was a real inducement.

CHAPTER SEVENTEEN

The restaurant was small and resonated with the owner's favorite Italian songs, which he sang in a shaky but enthusiastic baritone. Everyone applauded. It was filled with late customers, all of whom seemed to be relaxing after a long day. Jeff found us a table against the wall away from the loud speaker, and ordered us lasagna and beer. Both were welcome and delicious.

"Thanks for help with the surgery today," Jeff said, offering me a salty chip from a bowl on the table. "We were really shorthanded. Without your help, I'd have to postpone the surgery until tomorrow, and I'm not sure of the outcome with either the dog or the snake."

"I enjoyed it. In fact, I found it exciting."

He smiled. "I wasn't sure you could manage the snake."

"Neither was I. I never held a snake before. I actually didn't mind touching Twistie after the first few minutes. It…she wasn't slimy at all."

"Snakes aren't slimy, contrary to popular belief. You'll get used to handling the animals. It took me a while, too. Veterinary schools don't get you used to all the animals you treat."

"What animals do you treat routinely?"

"Mostly dogs and cats, of course. I delivered a little girl's hamster the other day. She was distraught at her pet's pain, but delighted when she left. Now she has three hamsters."

Being obstetrician to a hamster must definitely be a specialized skill! Jeff continued: "I've also treated, beside hamsters, gerbils, guinea pigs, skunks and even porcupines. But not many snakes until this snake breeder moved to Centerville. I had to really study snake anatomy in my medical books before attempting my first case."

"Why does this man raise snakes?" I asked Jeff. To me, the idea seemed unnerving.

"For treating snake bites, mainly. Venom is invaluable as serum. And people seem to covet snakeskin, for some damned reason. It's pretty awful, in my opinion, that garments are made from living creatures. Entire species of birds were wiped out for ladies' hats a few years back. Animals for food is another question. Much of it is barbaric." He hesitated. "I'm sorry, I seem to be doing a lot of talking. I do that when I unwind. Incidentally, I think you'll be a fine veterinarian. You have an air of competence and responsibility around our clinic. Avery thought so, too."

His words blew me away because I thought I was in the way and unhelpful on many occasions. But my tendency was to underrate my efforts. "I really love being in the clinic. And I enjoyed watching you in surgery today. I learned a lot."

He smiled, his eyes lighting up. "I love surgery. Now tell me what made you decide on veterinary medicine."

I actually told him about my bulimia. He seemed genuinely interested.

"Must have been a hard time, Amy. I've got to meet your Molly sometime. I'm in awe of animals which help humans, like guide dogs. They're uncanny. I'm convinced they have a sixth sense." Then he told me a story about a guide dog which had helped a patient: "Jason's father accompanied his son and other members of a boy scout troop on a week's trip to a lake in a distant mountainous area. It was especially significant to Jason because he was a biplegic, with braces on his legs. He was accompanied by a guide dog, Blackie, a gift of Canine Companions. Blackie was a faithful buddy, chaperoning Jason safely around the halls at school by gently pushing against his braces.

'After lunch one day the scouts decided to swim across a small river. Jason put on his life jacket, removed his leg braces, and entered the river, with Blackie happily following. Jason sank into the water and paddled along with his strong arms, but the current was more powerful than he'd expected and he was being tugged rapidly downstream. The other boys called to him but his nose had filled with water and he was panicking.

'Blackie had never been called on to save his master's life in water, but suddenly the dog was beside Jason, pushing against him as he did in school corridors. Jason grabbed his fur, and the dog pulled him safely to shore. On the beach, Jason hugged his exhausted dog, and realized that Blackie had saved his life, not only because it was his duty, but because Blackie loved him.'"

Amy looked into Jeff's face. "What a wonderful story," I said. "Animals are amazing. I wouldn't be here without Molly."

To my utter astonishment, Jeff took my hand, which was on the table, and kissed it. "Bless Mollie," he said. "I told you, I have to meet your Molly sometime. She sounds like a wonderful dog."

After dinner, I drove home feeling buoyant from my conversation with Jeff. My mother was still awake and my father was at the hospital. As we had done so often, my mother and I had a cup of tea. Molly licked my hand and curled up at my feet. I rumpled her neck and she put her head on my shoe and went to sleep.

"I had such a good time with Doctor Jeff," I told my mother. "He's one of the vets in the clinic. I don't know much about him, but he's a nice guy. He doesn't treat me like a lowly student even if I am one. He even let me watch him operate on a snake."

"A snake! Good heavens! I couldn't do it, Amy, but I'm glad you could. I'd be terrified."

"It wasn't bad at all, Mom. You just have to get used to it. My next snake won't be half as hard."

"Your next snake?" Mom shook her head. "You are fearless, my dear."

"I wish I were. Dad's at the hospital?"

"Delivering twins, no less."

I felt mischievous. "Did I tell you that Dr. Jeff delivered triplets?"

"Triplets? How on earth…?"

"Maybe I forget to mention that they were hamsters! They belong to a little girl. The hamster needed a Caesarian section."

Mom chuckled. "He sounds like a miracle worker."

"That's just what I called him."

Dad came home a half-hour later, looking tired but upbeat. "How'd it go?" Mom asked. I'd heard my mother ask the same concerned question hundreds of times when Dad returned from the hospital late at night.

Dad suppressed a yawn. "Very well. Mother and babies doing fine. The father's elated: he's handing out cigars to everyone including the cleaning crew. I've got three in my pocket right now." He held them up. "What have you two been up to?"

"I played bridge and Amy had dinner with her boss at the clinic," Mom said. "We both had a good time."

Dad looked at me. "What's happened to the Towns boy? The lawyer's son."

"A lot," I answered. "He's working in construction this summer. He's quit his law studies at the university and changed his major to history."

Dad seemed astonished "Good for him! Old Henry must be having a fit. At least he won't be bothering you anymore, Amy. Sounds as if his son has made up his own mind."

"I don't think I'll be hearing from Rod's father any more, Dad."

Dad patted me on the shoulder. "Good. Now I'm going to bed. See you all in the morning."

"We're coming, too," Mom said. And we all trooped up to our bedrooms, Molly following.

Next day, while I checked the kennels with Grace, she said, "I understand you assisted Dr. Jeff yesterday in surgery."

I nodded. "I even cleaned a snake. I still can't believe it, Grace."

Grace laughed. "Thanks for filling in, Amy; we were unexpectedly shorthanded."

"I really liked it. Dr. Jeff explained what he was doing during the entire surgery. It was very instructive."

"He helped me a lot when I was learning the routine here. He's not married so he has a little extra time to give to the practice and to tutor us. He comes in at the crack of dawn and often stays late. What wife would put up with that?"

"Not many, I'm sure."

Grace went on: "I asked him once. 'A good-looking man like you, you should get married,' I told him, just kidding. 'I never had the time,' he answered. 'A beginning veterinary practice takes more time than there is in a day.' There are three vets now so maybe there's more personal time for each of them."

I thought to myself, "Maybe I won't have much time, either, but I don't think I'll mind it because I'll love what I'm doing."

Ruth called at noon and said, "How about meeting for a quick lunch? Can you get away?"

"Sure. I found a new place right behind this clinic. Can you meet me there?"

She readily agreed, since the hospital is only a mile away.

She arrived promptly at noon. "This place is darling," she said, looking at the pictures of Enrico Caruso and the Tuscan countryside on the walls. "How did you ever find it?"

"I worked late last night and my boss took me here for a bite. It's not fancy but the food is great."

"It sounds as if things are going well at your veterinary clinic, Amy."

"They are. I even helped Jeff—that's Dr. Dubin—operate on a snake."

Her reaction was like Mom's. "A snake! How could you stand it?"

"It's gets easier when you're used to it. At least that's what Jeff says."

"Jeff? Is he a nice guy?"

I laughed. "Don't get the wrong idea, Ruth. This is a working relationship. All the vets are nice but Jeff is special because he's closer to my age. And he's helped me a lot. Have you seen Rod lately?"

Ruth looked at me, and her eyebrows rose. "That's a coincidence. Last night I saw him in town, and we grabbed a sandwich at the diner. He's doing some kind of project about the Middle Ages. He said to say 'hi.'"

"Has his father been pestering him?"

"I didn't ask, but I think he'd have told me if he was."

Ruth was already immersed in her university class on operating room techniques. On occasion she'd been asked to help the nurses prepare for surgery. "It's tough but interesting," she said. "Luckily, my patients aren't snakes."

"To each his own," I laughed.

"Let's do this again," Ruth said as their allotted lunch hours came to a close. "It's not far for me and I like your hideaway."

"Say hello to Rod. I don't get away from the clinic much so I haven't seen him."

"You know, he's a really nice guy. I'll tell him. Bye, Amy."

"So long, Ruth."

CHAPTER EIGHTEEN

For several days, I tended to the animals recovering from surgery, always under the supervisory eyes of the three vets. Twistie, the snake, had fully recovered, a dog with a broken leg had been splinted and gone home, a small dog recovering from bites inflicted by a German shepherd had been stitched up and would go home tomorrow, and a cat chased up a tree by a dog was being evaluated for treatment. Jeff explained, as Dr. Gregory had done in vet school, that a cat can easily climb a tree by digging in its curved claws, but often couldn't come down because its claws were not curved the right way. This cat had actually fallen from the tree as he tried to descend.

Naturally, Dr. Jeff oversaw the care of his animals as did Drs. McDonald and Stokes, but the feeding and superficial care was left to me. I changed dressings after surgery, walked dogs when they needed it, massaged the cat's back, and gave medicines at the allotted times. Sometimes Grace and I set up intravenous equipment for the doctors to use prior to surgery. I was learning fast.

"What prompted you to go into veterinary medicine?" I asked Jeff one day when I was observing him bandage a dog after surgery.

He continued taping the dog's wounds. "I had rheumatic fever as a kid. First I had a streptococcal infection, which kept me in bed almost a month, and then it was followed by the fever. Luckily, I didn't have heart involvement. But my dog, Lance, stayed by my bedside the entire time I was on bed rest, and took walks with me when I was recovering." He glanced at me and smiled. "Like you, a dog saved my life."

I helped Jeff to place a bell-shaped collar around the recovering dog's neck so he wouldn't tear at his wounds. "What happened to Lance?"

Jeff looked up from his bandaging. "He died like a trooper. My friends and I always went to the matinee at the movies every Saturday, walking up a long hill and descending on the other side into the small town where the movie theater was located. Lance followed us one day, happily tagging along. Like an idiot, I didn't see the danger. He couldn't come into the theatre with us so he waited patiently outside for us to come out. When we didn't, he wandered into the street and was hit and killed by a car. I will never forgive myself. He was a loyal little dog, and I suppose I've been trying to make it up to him ever since."

I could understand his grief. I have read story after story about people devastated by the illnesses and deaths of their pets, whether dogs, cats, hamsters…and maybe even snakes. One couple Grace told me about owned a Great Pyrenees for which they gave a birthday party every year. Every dog in the neighborhood was invited. Even the local cats liked the dog, and when it passed on, one still slept on his grave in the couple's backyard every warm night. Grace said the couple was still trying to recover from the loss of their beloved friend. Such is the devotion many have for their animals.

After clinic hours, Jeff turned to me. "How about another meal at the Italian restaurant? I don't feel like cooking."

No doubt about it, he was a bachelor. I jumped at the chance, because I enjoyed his company and appreciated his kindness to an inexperienced colleague. "Sounds great, Jeff."

"And, by the way, one day—I told you--I'd like to meet your Molly. She sounds like a great dog."

"I'm planning to bring her in." It made me inordinately happy that Jeff wanted to see my dog. This was a far different world for me from those terrible days when I stayed in bed and hoped to die. Working in the clinic was filled with busy days, but also with camaraderie in that we were all working with animals we cared about. I hoped it would never change.

Of course, we did have some strange dogs and not a few bizarre owners. These were light moments in the practice as well as desperate ones. One dog, a spotted spaniel, beloved by his master, was always well dressed for every occasion. He even arrived at the clinic attired in a vest and bowtie. When riding in the owner's convertible, the owner claimed, the dog wore custom goggles and a long silk scarf, which billowed in the wind. When the dog went skiing, it wore the goggles plus a custom ski jacket, and child-sized sneakers which fit into custom designed 42" skis! The dog's owner told Doctor McDonald that in the summer, the owner packed two duffel bags, one for his own equipment and the other containing gear for his dog. The dog's duffel contained towels, sunglasses, a bathing suit, and a custom-made life jacket for, the owner said, "those speedboat rides on the lake." In addition, he was provided with a special rubber jacket and oxygen tank, which fed into a clear plastic bubble fitted around the dog's head. "This way," the owner said, "we can explore the bottom of the lake. Rex really loves our adventures together."

"Do you believe that?" I asked Dr. McDonald. "What dog would put up with such nonsense?"

Dr. McDonald shrugged. "Who knows? Dogs can be trained to do remarkable things. But I never heard of a dog who could learn to ski, scuba dive, and required a bathing suit to swim."

I thought it totally ludicrous, but at least that man loved his dog and craved its companionship. The dog owners I couldn't abide were the ones who were cruel to their animals. Thankfully, they rarely came to our clinic.

One I won't forget came with his mixed breed Husky and wanted the dog put down. "I don't want to ever lay eyes on Rex again," he said angrily. I hate the animal."

Dr. Stokes was covering the practice that afternoon because Dr. McDonald was at a meeting and Jeff Dubin was assisting another nearby vet. Dr. Stokes rose to his full six foot four inch height. "But there's nothing wrong with the dog, Mr. McIntyre. Why do you want to put your dog down? Look at him; he's a handsome animal. He's got a beautiful coat, he's good natured, and…"

"You heard me, Doc? I don't ever want to see 'im again. He's no good an' I won't keep him. If'n you won't get rid of him, I'll get a gun and shoot him."

Dr. Stokes was shocked and I was speechless. I thought the man was crazy and might do something to all of us in his rage. Dr. Stokes clearly wasn't getting anywhere by trying to reason with this man. "But I can't put a healthy dog down, Mr. McIntire. It's illegal, for one thing, and for another, I don't want to do it. Why do you want to kill this animal?"

McIntyre's face contorted with anger and he actually gnashed his teeth. "All right, I'll tell ya since you don't git it. My wife, she divorced me. She tole me I could have the damn dog since I liked Rex so much. Well, I don't like him no more, and I ain't gonna look at him no longer, neither. "

Dr. Stokes tried desperately to keep his cool. I could see his fingers slowly clenching and unclenching. "Where does your wife live, Mr. McIntire? She won't take the dog?"

"I ain't gonna let her take him. I'll get rid of him, that'll show her. She lives in Brewster, far enough away so's the dog ain't gonna run to her. Now, you gonna get rid of Rex or you want me ta do it?"

Dr. Stokes grabbed Rex's leash from the furious owner. "I'll take him, Mr. McIntire. Don't give it a second thought."

"I ain't gonna. Good riddance." And he stalked from the clinic building, banging the door behind him.

I felt traumatized. Dr. Stokes rubbed Rex's ears and spoke to him calmly; in response, the dog wagged his tail. "One thing I'm not going to do," Dr. Stokes said," is put this dog down." He walked Rex to one of the outside pens, the dog following on the lead calmly and obediently. Then he turned to me. "Amy, see if you can find a McIntyre in the Brewster telephone book. It's only thirty miles away. Maybe we can locate the family."

There was no McIntyre in the Brewster phone book, but I figured that she might be a new resident, so I called Information. Sure enough, there was a Reba McIntyre living in the Brewster area. I found Dr. Stokes in his office and handed him the number. He motioned me to stay while he made the call.

Reba was overjoyed to get Dr. Stokes' call. When he explained that Rex was in the care of the clinic, and how that had occurred, I could hear her happy voice from where I stood. "I'll drive right over," she said. "Give me an hour. He's a wonderful dog and I can't wait to get him back."

Sure enough, within an hour she was hugging Rex and thanking Dr. Stokes for returning her dog. "I'm so happy to have him," she said. "My children and I love him so much. I can't tell you how we missed him."

She offered to pay Dr. Stokes but he wouldn't take the money. Instead, he beamed at the prospect of Rex's return to a family which loved him. I realized that owners can be cruel and ignorant sometimes and that I'd never get used to it.

I told Jeff about it that night at dinner in the Italian restaurant. "Good for Warren," Jeff said. "I hate to put a dog down, too, even if it's sick. But definitely not a lovely, healthy animal like Rex."

I thought about his words. "But what do you do when the owners deny that their dogs are sick and you know that they're suffering?"

"Even if it's inhumane," Jeff said, "it's the owner's choice. Recently an owner came in with a dog which had tried to attack an SUV head-on. The animal ended up badly mangled. When I tried to convince the owner that her dog should be put down, she kept insisting that the dog was just a little "grubby" but would be fine tomorrow. I tried to tell her that the dog would die in terrible pain, but she countered that 'he just needed to be taken for a nice walk.' When the dog died a few breaths later, I think she blamed me, and when she fainted, we had to call an ambulance." He shook his head. "Some owners are in complete denial, and I feel sorry for them, but sometimes I can't do anything to convince them."

I shoved my food around my plate, barely able to eat. "It's so sad. I know how I'd feel if I lost Molly."

He nodded and changed the subject. "Which reminds me: when can I see your wonder dog?"

Again I was flattered and laughed at his wish to see my dog. "I'll bring her to work tomorrow."

"Good! She'll be comfortable in that empty pen out back and you can take her for walks during the day."

"Thanks, Jeff."

"By the way, when do you go back to vet school, Amy?"

"Three weeks." I felt suddenly sad at the thought. "This summer has gone too fast. I can hardly believe it's almost over."

"For me, too. It's been nice having you with us. Would you like to come back for vacations and next summer as an intern? I've already spoken about it with Avery and Warren. They absolutely agree with me. We all want you back."

It took my breath away. An internship? "You mean it?"

He nodded. "Of course I mean it."

I could barely talk. "I'd absolutely love it," I said. What a great, unexpected prospect! "Th..thanks," I managed to stammer. I'd learned so much this summer, and had grown even more in love with the profession, that I could hardly believe that the vets felt the same way about me. I was happier than I'd felt in a long while. His arm on the table was resting against mine, and I felt exhilarated by the feel of it. Molly had brought about a miracle; I hoped it would continue forever.

I told my parents when I reached home, that I had been invited to be an intern at the clinic during vacations. "Jeff Dubin told me today," I said. "I know that he's probably most responsible for asking me to continue at the clinic because I work most closely with him. But the other men agreed."

My father had just returned from the hospital and had settled with his newspaper into his favorite armchair. I sat on the couch opposite. "Congratulations," he said as he dropped his newspaper to look over at me. "You must have done really well, Amy. I'm proud of you."

"Thanks, Dad."

My mother was sewing. She dropped it into her lap to listen to me. She had a big smile on her face. "It's wonderful to have a job lined up for next summer," she said. "I hear that many people don't. Your Dr. Dubin sounds very nice, Amy."

"He is. He's been a good teacher. A friend, too. He wants to meet Molly tomorrow," I said. "I've bragged about her so often that Jeff calls her a miracle dog." When I mentioned her name, Molly wagged her tail as if she knew what I was saying. I rubbed her glossy coat while she contentedly leaned against my leg.

"She's really special," my mother agreed. "He'll see that as soon as he lays eyes on her."

It dawned on me that I hadn't seen Ruth and Rod in a couple of weeks. Tomorrow, I thought, I'll call. For now, I needed to pile into bed. So I did, with Molly cuddling beside me.

CHAPTER NINETEEN

Ruth was celebrating the end of nursing exams when I called her at home. I knew that her summer courses had kept her cloistered.

"What are you doing?" I ask her. "Something exciting, I hope."

"Cleaning the silver. Mom's having a dinner party. Want to come over and help?"

"Thanks anyway for your generous offer," I laugh. "No offense, but I'd rather clean the bathroom."

She whooped. "I figured."

"Ruth, isn't there something we can do to celebrate the end of your exams besides clean house? I have good news, too."

"Great idea! Let's have dinner tonight at The Pub. I'll ask Rod. I drive home right past his construction site." It seems that we always celebrate happy events at The Pub, but that's all we can afford, and, besides, it's centrally located, it's cozy, and the food is good.

"Great. I haven't seen either of you in a blue moon. He's doing all right?"

"Says he is. Tonight at 6?"

"See you then."

I arrive first, order a glass of wine, and read the menu while I wait for my friends. Italian dishes always make my mouth water: manicotti, tortellini, spaghetti with marinara sauce, meatballs.

I was trying to make a decision when Ruth and Rod walked in.

Rod was sunburned from working outside on his construction job, and Ruth looked relaxed and smiling after her exams. She'd pulled her hair back from her face and tied it into a ponytail with a bright ribbon. Tonight she looked especially festive and pretty.

"Long time no see," I exclaim as she and Rod arrive at my table. "I think we've all been hibernating."

"Sure feels like it," Ruth agrees. "Thank heavens exams are over."

She makes a hallelujah gesture with both arms raised skyward. "It's like getting out of jail."

I know the feeling exactly. "How'd they go, Ruth?"

"Not bad. Pretty good, actually."

I could have predicted that result because Ruth always aces her exams. "How about you, Rod?" In contrast to Ruth, he seems pretty subdued. He's got a day's growth of beard, which could be that he didn't have time to shave, or he's trying to be "one of the guys" on the building site. At any rate, it looks pretty good, rugged and manly.

"It's going okay except my father's driving me crazy. He cruises past my work site every damned day to check on me, then parks his Mercedes by the side of the road and watches. All the other workmen have noticed him, too, and wonder why he just sits there. So I told them what was going on, and to ignore him But that's not easy when he's staring at me for an hour every day."

"He hopes he'll intimidate you enough so you'll return to law school," I tell him, as if he hasn't figured it out already. "In the meantime, he wants to make sure you're uncomfortable."

"Well, he's succeeding." Rod's voice echoes his disgust.

"But you won't return, will you?" Ruth asks, sounding concerned. "Your dad's just acting like a jerk. You won't let him influence you, will you?"

Rod hits his fist on the table. "Not on your life. I've got a year as a history major and another as an assistant practicing classroom teaching. I've made my decision."

Ruth looks relieved, then glances across the table at me. "What's going on at your clinic, Amy?"

My news pales with the problems Rod is having, but I barge ahead anyway. "Jeff Dubin, one of our vets, has asked me to return as an intern during vacations this year, and then next summer." I can't keep the excitement out of my voice. "I still can't believe it."

"Congratulations!" Ruth exclaims. "You're so lucky!"

"Don't I know it!"

Rod chimes in, "Your clinic must really like you, Amy. Jobs are scarce right now. Everybody's looking and not having much luck.

"What about you, Ruth?" I ask. "I've heard jobs are available for nurses because hospitals in this area are advertising in the paper."

She crosses her fingers and nods. "I hope."

We order from our Italian waiter, who can barely speak English, but we manage to communicate by pointing to the menu and using hand signals. While we're waiting to be served, Ruth asks, "Do you like the docs you're working for, Amy?"

"They're all great. I brought Molly over to the clinic this morning so Dr. Dubin could admire her. I told him about my bulimia and he calls her a wonder dog. He talked to her whenever he passed her outdoor pen and gave her a dog biscuit. I'll bring her home when I leave here."

Ruth laughs. "Sounds as if Molly and your doctor speak the same language."

"I'm sure they do. Some people have a way with animals. Dr. Dubin is one of them."

"What's amazing to me," Rod breaks in, "is that vets see so many different kinds of animals with different anatomies, temperaments, and habits. How can they possibly treat snakes, hamsters, rabbits, dogs, and cats in one day?"

"To say nothing of the temperaments of all their owners," Ruth agrees. "I've seen women take their pets for walks in doll carriages at the mall while others let their pets bark and snarl at passersby."

I've seen these pets, too. "Some of the animals brought into our clinic are terrors and others obey their owners. Last week an owner, a big assertive woman with strong opinions, brought in a cat weighing twenty-five pounds in a large, fancy cage with wheels like a suitcase and "Baby" printed on the sides. She talked baby talk to the cat and called it 'her little darling sweetie.' When she saw Dr. Stokes putting on gloves to remove the cat from the cage, she was insulted. 'You're a veterinarian and afraid of my little kitty?' she blustered. 'Why, she's a pussycat.' She glared at Dr. Stokes with a look that could kill. 'I'll get my baby out for you,' she said coldly.

"As she reached into the cage, we heard a snarl, a scream, and the woman came out with a bloody hand and arm. 'Help,' she wailed, 'help me. Don't just stand there, I need help!' Dr. Stokes promptly slammed the cage door shut until the "darling kitty" calmed down; then he removed it from its cage and proceeded to treat it.

"Meanwhile, Grace and another technician took the hysterical woman, who was shrieking that Dr. Stokes had upset her normally sweet-tempered little kitty, into an adjacent examining room to bandage her wounds. When Grace tried to point out that it was the owner herself who handled the cat, not Dr. Stokes, she wouldn't listen. Incidentally, she never paid for either her own or the cat's care."

Ruth was visibly shocked. "I'm glad at least that it wasn't your Dr. Stokes who was injured."

"So am I."

Amazingly, just as we're finishing our meal, I look up and there is Jeff Dubin walking into the restaurant with an attractive woman about thirty years old holding his arm in a proprietary way. He appears as astonished as I am.

"Amy!" he says. "What a surprise!"

"You, too, Jeff," I answer, feeling momentarily off-balance. I introduce Jeff and his guest to my friends. "Ruth Schofield and Rod Towns, this is Dr. Jeff Dubin. Jeff is a veterinarian at the clinic where I work".

Jeff extends his hand. "My sister, Mary. She's visiting for a few days." While I'm adjusting to the revelation that this attractive woman is Jeff's sister and not a fiance´ or friend, he turns to me. "Do you come here often?"

"It's our favorite place, Jeff." Then I explain to Rod and Ruth about the restaurant behind the clinic. "We'll have to meet there next time. Jeff introduced me to it." It's obvious to Rod and Ruth by now that Jeff's a friend as well as my boss. I'm happy about it.

"Listen, thanks for bringing Molly to the clinic today," Jeff says. "She's an awfully nice dog."

"Thanks. I know she is. She's so full of dog biscuits that she'll never leave the clinic."

"By the way," Jeff says, "I've got some gloomy news. That puppy mill or one like it is back in our area. Avery thinks it's the same one because of the type of wounds he's treating. They're selling their dogs just outside town, but they change location so often that they're hard to track down. The cops are trying to locate where the dogs come from so they haven't arrested the sellers yet. One of the cops called Avery at the office to warn him."

Jeff looks at Rod and Ruth. "Are you Amy's friends who helped her find the last puppy mill?"

Rod nods. "It was a miserable place. I never saw anything like it. I mean it; it was pathetic. The police knew where it was located so we could find it. I hope they locate this one."

"But isn't there something we can do?" I ask Jeff.

He shakes his head. "These people are dangerous and they're committing a felony. I warn you, don't try to find them—that warning comes from the police. You could get hurt. These people are criminals and they're protecting their business. Besides, the sheriff's office is already on the case. These crooks could retaliate. Only warning the public would help."

When Jeff and his sister leave for their table near us, we look at each other, puzzled, because we don't know what to do. We've seen what these people do to torture animals, and can't stand to see other animals held against their will under similar circumstances. But would they get even with humans who got in their way?

"They don't have any human feelings," Rod says, as we remembered the Sidwells declaring that their dogs didn't have feelings. "It's dangerous."

"Then where does that leave us?" Ruth asks. "What can we do?"

Rod thinks it over. "I still know that cop. He'll tell us when he finds out where they keep the dogs."

"But we can't just barge in, like last time," Ruth says. "Dr. Dubin says it's dangerous and I believe him."

"A newspaper article?" Amy asks.

Rod nods. "Maybe."

"Then I'll write the article," I tell them. "That's something I can do. If Jeff's worried, I'll use a fictitious name."

"Then use my name," Rod says. "If they accept the article, we could leave copies at stores around town to warn potential buyers."

There's no way I'm going to use Rod's name, but using a fictitious name sounds like a possibility. I'll go home tonight, write the article, show it to Jeff, and submit it.

Jeff and his sister are still at their table, so I mention it to him as we're leaving.

"You've got more courage than a tiger," Jeff says. " No, we'll use my name because the clinic is involved. I admire your determination, Amy, but it's my legal responsibility. I should have seen that all along."

When I relate Jeff's decision to Rod and Ruth, Rod agrees. "It is Dr. Dubin's responsibility, Amy. But we can all help by distributing copies of the paper if they publish your article. That way, we'll all be doing something."

"When the police know where the puppy mill is located," Ruth says, "we can inform the local animal shelter. They'd know how to place the dogs with good owners."

It's a good decision. In my article, I'll try to describe the conditions we saw at the puppy farm. Most people don't even know about puppy farms, or if they do, they don't know what to do about them. My article will tell them about the horrific conditions these dogs must endure, about the tiny cages they live in, forced to have endless puppies when all they want is human companionship and a little kindness. Maybe we can convince enough people to join with us in our determination to shut it down.

On my way home, I'm already composing my article.

CHAPTER TWENTY

I worked until after 2 in the morning to write the article for the newspaper. Once I got started, I couldn't stop. Molly sat beside my chair, wagged her tail, and gave me strength. I petted her neck, told her what a good dog she was, and tried to imagine her in that breeder's care, which only served to fuel my indignation. I found it impossible to describe to anyone who had not seen it, the filth, stench, and desperate cries of the imprisoned animals, the maimed dogs we saw, the endless spinning of the dogs gone cage-crazy. I wanted to vomit, trying to describe it and feared that my bulimia might return again. My stomach ached as it hadn't in months. I forced myself to stay in front of my computer and not move until I had at least finished an outline, but by then I was so angry that I continued.

I wrote about the injured animals which had lost limbs because they were so weak from lack of exercise and good food that they broke bones when they were put down on solid ground. I had seen these animals in our clinic, and knew how desperate and unhealthy they were.

I described the dogs fixed by the breeders so they couldn't bark by sticking some kind of scissors down their throats to sever their vocal chords.

I remembered the nervous tics so many of the dogs exhibited from having spent so many years in cages.

I warned prospective buyers of breeders who had no credentials but nevertheless advertised on the Internet with glowing accounts of their dogs for sale. I mentioned that it was the spent and exhausted dogs, which had been bred repeatedly, that were sold to buyers, and that some had been caged for years and never allowed to walk on solid ground. I felt that I had to let the public know.

I had already learned from exploration on the Internet that the United States Department of Agriculture was supposed to enforce all animal welfare standards, including oversight of that puppy mill we had found in the woods. Even though the owner said that the USDA had given that horrible place an A rating, I was sure that no one from the USDA had even seen the site or cared about the fate of the tortured dogs. If a dog has food and water, I read that legally it could be locked in a cage for years without the owners being charged with animal abuse. The animals had no official representation. I discovered that Humane societies, local police, and groups like Petfinder.com and Save-a-Pet and Best Friends filled the gap as best they could, but most often the animals were left to the cruelty of unscrupulous and uncaring people. I poured all of my pent-up fury into my article, knowing that the editor would undoubtedly scrap half, if not all, of it. So why not tell him the truth and hope that someone on the staff cared about animals?

In the morning I pulled myself from bed, reread the article, printed it and put it in a folder to hand to Jeff. I was still full of anger and indignation at the plight of animals when I walked into the clinic. But to my chagrin, Jeff wasn't there. Grace informed me that he had gone to treat a sick dog, then on to attend a noon meeting of the county veterinary society and might be back in the late afternoon, or not at all.

I thought of all those sick dogs crying for release from their cages or yearning for a single ray of sunshine let into their desperate lives, and I felt added urgency. I didn't want to wait a moment longer. So on my noon hour, I took my article to the newspaper office, handed it to the editor's secretary, a middle-aged woman who sat outside the editor's office.

"Nobody signed this article," she said, looking up at me. "Sorry, but we don't take unsigned letters."

"This isn't a letter," I said. "It's really a news story about a puppy mill near here."

She looked it over quickly. "It's opinion," she said "It's not an editorial so it's considered a letter."

"Would it help if a veterinarian at the clinic signed it?" I asked.

"Not if you wrote it," she answered.

I didn't have much choice. "Then I'll sign it," I said.

I signed the letter and left it in the hands of people who I hoped could help. Then I left the building, knowing that Jeff couldn't sign the article so it had been my decision. I felt good that I'd made it. The secretary was reading my article as I left so at least someone would read it.

I ran into Jeff just as I returned to the clinic, and told him what I'd done. "I signed it, Jeff, because they wouldn't take it without my signature."

He put his hand to his forehead. "Damn, I didn't think of that."

"Don't worry, they probably won't even print it."

"Whether they do or not, I'm going to call the police. I don't want to take any chance on what that creep at the puppy mill might or might not do. I want to get those dogs under protection immediately."

"Have any more dogs come into the clinic?"

He nodded. "Avery just got one. It's got worms, is underweight, and her coat is matted and filthy. Avery took one look and knew exactly where it came from."

"But why did the woman buy the dog if it looked so bad?"

"She told Avery, "Jeff explained, "that she was driving and saw a "Puppies For Sale" sign by the road. She had volunteered once in an animal shelter, and had some knowledge of what she was witnessing. Her curiosity was aroused so she stopped her car to look at the dozen or so dogs enclosed in a pen. As she approached, the dogs started crying and baying pathetically, and one was jumping up and down frantically trying to attract her attention. "You can have any of 'em for ten dollars," the woman said, "'cause we're gonna put 'em all down."

"But these dogs are perfectly healthy," the drive-by woman protested. "You can't kill these animals. It's callous and not even legal."

"They're no damn good to me," the dog owner had declared vehemently, "Why should I keep feeding no-good animals?"

The drive-by woman had stared at the owner, trying to fathom how anyone could be so heartless about these dogs in her care. It absolutely had to be the Sidwells at work.

"Then I'll take that one," the drive-by lady had said, pointing to the little white female which had been so desperately trying to attract her attention. She told me she'd planned to bring the dog to the Humane Society to find it a good home but then she fell in love with it herself."

Jeff went on in a solemn voice: "That little dog had never felt grass before, sat on furniture, played with a toy, or known human affection. The woman brought the animal to our clinic for treatment. It only had a number, tattooed inside its ear, undoubted inflicting great pain on the unsuspecting animal. What have I done to deserve this, the little dog must have thought. The new owner promptly named the little dog Lucky, and she truly is a lucky little dog."

I was anxious to meet Lucky, so asked Jeff to show me where she'd been placed.

He led me to the back of the clinic, where a bed had been made for her in an isolation pen. At the clinic, she had been bathed, examined, and inoculated with required shots. The poor animal was gaunt and bony. When I put my hand inside the pen to pet it, the little dog tentatively moved closer and then licked her. "Give it a few more days and you'll see a different dog," Jeff said. "She's on the road to recovery."

I wanted to pet Lucky longer, but held off until tomorrow because she looked exhausted; her day had been filled with incredible challenges, but she was safe. If she could survive her mistreatment, her life in the future would be unlike anything she'd experienced in the past.

The next morning, I was barely awake when my parents knocked on my bedroom door. When I answered, they rushed in holding the morning newspaper. Unbelievably, my article was at the bottom of the front page. Without a word, they held it out for me to read. I could hardly believe it. My Dad said with a chuckle, "Maybe the owner of the next puppy mill that comes along will think twice before settling here."

"They'd better," my Mom agreed. "Now everyone will know how those people treat their dogs and no one will buy them. They're such miserable characters, so inhumane."

Dad nodded in agreement. "Are they any danger to the clinic, Amy? Or, my God, to you?"

I shook my head, trying to convey an assurance I didn't entirely feel. "Dr. McDonald has already called the police. He told them he didn't want those crooks taking revenge on the clinic or its employees."

"But you wrote the article," Dad said. "You're the one they'd take it out on."

I knew that Dr. McDonald was taking every precaution. "The police said they'd station a patrolman in the neighborhood, just in case. But they think the article will scare the owners of the dogs out of town. And the police will be right on their tail."

"But what will happen to the dogs?" Mom asked.

"Jeff said that the Humane Society will take as many as they can manage and transfer the rest to other societies. They'll need a lot of rehabilitation. I'd like to go see them when they're settled."

"I'll go with you," Mom said. "If they need petting, I'm available. And I hope those people at the puppy mill land in jail."

Dad nodded. "And the jailors throw away the key."

"I'm sure they will," I answered, feeling more confident, "when the police see the condition of the animals."

"You bet," Mom replied. "After all, lots of cops own dogs, too."

CHAPTER TWENTY-ONE

Dr. McDonald calls a meeting in his office that morning, with Drs. Stokes, Jeff Dubin, and myself attending. "I don't think those people will cause us any trouble," Dr. McDonald says. "The police know where they are, which is heading out of town with their dogs crammed into two big trucks. They can't hide very easily so the police are rounding them up as we speak. I'm afraid we'll be inundated with sick dogs for a while because I've volunteered this clinic to donate time and effort to treat the animals. Other vets in the area are also helping out." He looks around. "I hope you all agree."

Dr. Stokes and Jeff nod solemnly.

Dr. McDonald continues. "Thanks, Amy, for getting everyone stirred up with that article in the paper. I've had phone calls since dawn from people volunteering their services to care for the animals until they can be adopted. Many of them didn't even know what a puppy mill was! Now they do."

I'm bowled over by Dr. McDonald's praise and by the words of the others as we leave the office. Grace pats me on the arm. "I knew you'd be an asset to this clinic, Amy. It'll be nice to work with you in the future." She even gives me a hug.

"Thanks, Grace. Can I see Lucky today?"

"Of course. She's doing a little better." Grace leads me into the isolation area where the little dog is eating a special diet of wholesome grains, meats and vegetables for weight gain. I know she hasn't had a decent meal in recent months, if ever. It's a joyful experience to watch her eat; now and then she even wags her tail. At least they hadn't cut it off in their calculated butchery.

As soon as I return to the office, my cell phone started ringing, first from Ruth, then Rod. " I'm so glad we discovered that first puppy mill," Ruth says. "That's what started the ball rolling against those dog owners. But it was your letter that really did it."

"No, it was the three of us, Ruth. We did it together. We're the three musketeers, remember?"

Ruth laughs. "Of course. Movies tonight, to celebrate?"

"Great idea."

"I'll ask Rod."

Jeff finds me in the supply room where I'm restocking some of our medications. "Amy, thanks again for going ahead with that letter. I'm sorry you couldn't find me. It was a great letter and got lots of needed attention. Now readers will be on the lookout for puppy mills and abused animals."

I feel happy in his praise. "I didn't think it would work out so well."

"Neither did I. By the way, when do you go back to school?"

I'd barely thought of school, with so much going on at the clinic. "In three weeks, Jeff. But I'll be back for fall break. I'll count each day."

"So will I, Amy."

My heart skips a beat and I look at him searchingly. Was that just a casual comment or did he mean something more? I'd admired Jeff ever since I came to the clinic for his kindness, skill, and devotion to our animals. He's a fine veterinarian, but does he care about me--a student, a beginner, and low woman on the totem pole? I doubted it. Yet he'd stood up for me when Rod, Ruth and I found the puppy mill. He'd let me help in his surgery. He'd encouraged me when I needed help with the animals or with clinic procedures. I always knew he was there to help if I needed him.

But he was continuing. "Amy, I'll be coming to the university in about a month to take a weekend refresher on new techniques and to see some old colleagues. Will you have a free day? Maybe we could go hiking, have dinner, or see a game..."

I'm bowled over. "That would be fun, Jeff!" I don't even hesitate. "I'd love to spend the day with you." I'd used my time at school mostly studying, and at home, writing about disgusting people who torture dogs. There are lots better things in life, I've told myself, and being friends with Jeff was definitely one of them.

I'm feeling upbeat when I meet Ruth and Rod. "That was a great article in the paper," Rod says. "The cops tell me that the police have located the puppy-mill trucks heading out of town."

"Good riddance!" Ruth exclaims. "I hope that prison is their next destination."

"I'm sure of it," Rod answers.

I feel strongly about it, too. "I can't bear to think of all the dogs they've tortured. The doctors in the clinic have volunteered to treat many of them so some can be returned to a happy existence.

"They deserve it," Rod agrees. "Nothing can make up for what those animals have suffered."

We talk about returning to the university. "I've saved up enough money to pay for the fall semester and for part of my classes in the spring," Rod says. "My foreman said he'd rehire me any time I'm home, which means over Christmas. Mom says I can stay at the house over the holidays."

I'm surprised. "She does? But what about your Dad?"

"Mom says he can grumble all he wants, to ignore him. She says that's what she does when he gets in one of his moods."

We're amazed at the idea of the blustering Henry Towns under the control of his petite wife. He seems to me like a spoiled child, needing someone to challenge him. Good for Mrs. Towns to stand up to her bullying husband!

"It'll work out," Ruth says to Rod in a confident voice. "I'm sure it will."

After a walk down the main street of Centerville, we end up at the movie theatre. I'm sitting next to Ruth when I notice Rod take her hand and hold it. It blows me away. I can't concentrate on the movie.

I hadn't known how they felt about each other. They have become my best friends and, momentarily, I feel alienated. Yet, sitting there beside her in that dark theater, I feel happy for Ruth, and for Rod, too. Besides, I'm developing a friendship with Jeff, so our lives may continue to touch each other.

I reflect that we were drawn together over our mutual love of animals, and that was a special kind of bond. We hated the torture that some humans inflicted on animals. I had laughed at the quotation ascribed to Andy Rooney, the television personality, who said, "The average dog is a nicer person than the average person."

I think people are kind to animals especially when they've been educated about them. If they knew of the incredible pain a cat feels when being declawed, having the delicate nerves severed and destroying his balance as well as his ability to defend himself, maybe they wouldn't have the procedure performed. I flinch when I see animal fur worn by humans who, I'm certain, never stopped to consider that their vanity came at the death of a living creature.

A woman who read my article in the paper sent me a quotation ascribed to Paul Harvey, the radio personality, who dearly loved animals:

I do not mean to suggest that it is but one step from
suffocating animals to putting people in ovens.
It's not.
It is several steps.
The first step begins with tolerating any pain which we cannot
ourselves feel.
Anguish is anguish. It knows no gender, no race, no species.

Harvey continued:

When it comes to suffering, the only thing separating the smartest of
us
from the dumbest of them is our vocal cords.
If we allow them to hurt only because they cannot speak,
May God have mercy on them—and us.

I have framed these words and placed them on the wall in my
school dorm. Next to Harvey's poems is one by William Blake, the
eighteenth century English poet:
Robin redbreast in a cage
Puts all of heaven in a rage.

****

I have almost finished my veterinary school studies, and continue
with a close relationship to Jeff, as does Ruth with Ron, who is working
hard on his Ph.D in history. We are still the three musketeers. Life goes
on happily for us, but for millions of animals in this country, life is
torture. Luckily, millions of people also love and protect them. Bless
their efforts.

Molly continues to live with us, provides us with affection, loves
long hikes, and is our guardian (or thinks she is). I still can't believe
my good luck in having her.